Personalizing Psychotherapy

Personalizing Psychotherapy

Assessing and Accommodating Patient Preferences

John C. Norcross
Mick Cooper

 AMERICAN PSYCHOLOGICAL ASSOCIATION

Published by
American Psychological Association
750 First Street, NE
Washington, DC 20002
https://www.apa.org

Order Department
https://www.apa.org/pubs/books
order@apa.org

In the U.K., Europe, Africa, and the Middle East, copies may be ordered from Eurospan
https://www.eurospanbookstore.com/apa
info@eurospangroup.com

Typeset in Charter and Interstate by Circle Graphics, Inc., Reisterstown, MD

Printer: Gasch Printing, Odenton, MD
Cover Designer: Gwen J. Grafft, Minneapolis, MN

Library of Congress Cataloging-in-Publication Data

Names: Norcross, John C., 1957- author. | Cooper, Mick, author.
Title: Personalizing psychotherapy : assessing and accommodating patient
    preferences / by John C. Norcross and Mick Cooper.
Description: Washington, DC : American Psychological Association, [2021] |
    Includes bibliographical references and index.
Identifiers: LCCN 2020037955 (print) | LCCN 2020037956 (ebook) |
    ISBN 9781433834554 (paperback) | ISBN 9781433834561 (ebook)
Subjects: LCSH: Psychotherapy. | Psychotherapist and patient.
Classification: LCC RC475 .N67 2021 (print) | LCC RC475 (ebook) |
    DDC 616.89/14—dc23
LC record available at https://lccn.loc.gov/2020037955
LC ebook record available at https://lccn.loc.gov/2020037956

https://doi.org/10.1037/0000221-000

Printed in the United States of America

10 9 8 7 6 5 4 3 2

To our integrative teachers and mentors:
James Prochaska, Marvin Goldfried, and John McLeod

Contents

Preface

To know what you prefer, instead of humbly saying Amen to what the world tells you ought to prefer, is to have kept your soul alive.

—Robert Louis Stevenson

Since its beginnings, psychotherapy has sought to adapt or fit itself to the individual patient. As early as 1919, Freud introduced psychoanalytic psychotherapy as an alternative to classical psychoanalysis on the recognition that the latter, more rarified approach lacked universal applicability and that many patients did not profit from or prefer it (Wolitzky, 2011). The mandate for individualizing psychotherapy is embodied in Gordon Paul's (1967) iconic question: "What treatment, by whom, is most effective for this individual with that specific problem, and under which set of circumstances?" (p. 111). Every psychotherapist recognizes that what works for one person may not work for another; we seek "different strokes for different folks" (Blatt & Felsen, 1993).

Hundreds of potential client characteristics have been proposed as markers for using one treatment method or relationship style rather than another (Clarkin & Levy, 2004). However, it has been only in the past 15 or 20 years that the quest for personalizing psychotherapy has been fully supported by solid research. The enshrined clinical lore of creating a new psychotherapy for each patient now rightfully carries the designation of *evidence-based practice*.

We focus in this volume on personalizing psychotherapy to client preferences. Why preferences? First, because doing so is a powerful way of communicating respect and valuing to clients, that their views matter and are worthy of consideration. We thus move from a paternalistic model of care toward a more democratic and collaborative one that acknowledges the centrality of client choice and expertise. Second, it brings to the fore the client's hopes, desires, and directions, rather than their disorders and pathologies. It asks the quintessentially human question "What do you want?" rather than "What is wrong with you?" Third, personalizing psychotherapy is associated with greater patient engagement and improved treatment outcomes. Fourth, patient preferences and values are clearly identified as one of the three sources of evidence-based practice. Fifth, honoring preferences embraces individual differences and actualizes cultural diversity. Sixth, students and patients highly value this method of individualizing treatment. Finally, there has yet to be a practical and applied guide to working with client preferences, despite the rapid growth of research in this field (Swift et al., 2019). Stated simply, understanding and valuing patient preferences prove human, collaborative, effective, popular, and necessary to clinical practice.

A warm welcome, then, to *Personalizing Psychotherapy: Assessing and Accommodating Patient Preferences*.

OUR AIM

In this book, we highlight evidence-based methods to gauge, honor, and implement client preferences in counseling and psychotherapy. We, the authors, are two seasoned scientist–practitioners on separate continents joined by our commitment to meeting clients where they are at and valuing their preferred ways of working. We strive to honor clients' preferences while also honoring our own expertise and understandings. By the end of this volume, we trust that you will be able to reliably determine a client's preferences and accommodate them when clinically and ethically indicated so that psychotherapy is personalized for each patient.

We aim in this volume to familiarize you with the empirical and clinical evidence for accommodating patient preferences in Chapters 1 through 3 and then to walk you through its clinical assessment and application in Chapters 4 through 9. The content of this book is about two-thirds application and one-third theory and research; more "how to" than "how come."

We begin in Chapter 1 by featuring the evolution of treatment adaptations or responsiveness, including the confusing multiplicity of terms for the process of creating a new psychotherapy for each patient. The next two chapters summarize the research evidence and clinical rationale, respectively, for personalizing to preferences. Then, in Chapters 4 and 5, we drill down to assessing client preferences and applying our favored instrument, the Cooper–Norcross Inventory of Preferences (C-NIP), as well as other measures. How to sensitively integrate preferences into psychotherapy is the focus of the next chapter, then training and supervision in Chapter 7. The book concludes by presenting the contraindications of personalizing in Chapter 8 and its probable (and exciting) directions in Chapter 9. We envision a more ethical, effective, and evidence-based bespoke psychotherapy in the future.

Throughout, we showcase numerous case examples from our clinical practices, supervisees' work, and research studies. In all cases, we have either obtained permission from the clients to audio record and present their words, constructed composite patients to disguise their identities and maintain their privacy, or both.

OUR AUDIENCES

Our intended audiences are psychotherapy and counseling practitioners, students, and trainers across the continents, of all persuasions and professions. We have strong reason to believe that most mental health professionals already individualize their work to some extent, but not as consistently, comprehensively, or effectively as possible.

We are not teaching here a particular treatment approach; instead, we build on your clinical competencies and favored theories. We are decidedly integrative (Norcross & Goldfried, 2019) and pluralistic (Cooper & McLeod, 2011) in our own orientation. To paraphrase Isaac Newton, we intend to build bridges, not walls. The book primarily focuses on psychotherapy with adult clients and on a one-to-one basis. However, we believe that those working with children and young people, as well as in groups or more community settings, will find much of value to take into their work.

Psychotherapy students will, we trust, find this pantheoretical, research-supported personalizing approach effective in practice and resonating in spirit. Most of us were attracted to the healing professions in order to nurture fellow souls qua individuals, not to provide manualized protocols to diagnostic "entities." Personalizing psychotherapy capitalizes on both the nomothetic and idiographic traditions: attuning psychotherapy to the particulars of the individual according to the generalities of the research.

As psychotherapy teachers ourselves, we believe that trainers and supervisors will find this volume helpful. It operationalizes what we all, repeatedly, preach: Treat the entire person, not only the diagnosis. It is a quintessentially whole-person approach to mental health services.

OUR WORD CHOICES

Throughout this book, we intentionally alternate the terms *patient* and *client* and use them interchangeably. The same applies to *psychotherapy*, *counseling*, and *treatment*, and we use the terms *psychotherapist*, *counselor*, and *clinician* interchangeably too. It is a matter not only of remaining theoretically pluralistic on these contentious word choices but also of communicating inclusivity across disciplines and traditions. When we speak of the *individual*, we naturally recognize that the person may be in individual therapy or in a larger treatment format, such as a couple or in a group.

We tend to privilege in clinical practice the terms and roles the patient favors, as opposed to what the psychotherapist desires. Wilfred Bion (1967), the famed psychoanalyst, meant something along these lines when he wrote about conducting therapy without memories and desires because they interfere and distort the client's lived experience. That is part and parcel of this book's meta-message: It is the patient's experiences and preferences that can, and should frequently, drive the work.

OUR ACKNOWLEDGMENTS

It takes a village to construct an assessment tool, such as the C-NIP, and to compile a book, such as this. We are indebted to scores of colleagues, students, patients, and collaborators. Particular gratitude is expressed to Jake S. Ziede and Danielle Cook for conducting literature reviews and chasing articles, Thomas P. Hogan for statistical expertise on the C-NIP and its development, and Gina di Malta for her collaboration on a wide range of related projects. We are grateful to Brett Raymond-Barker for gathering data on the use of the C-NIP, as well as Sarah Knox, Hanne Oddli, and Joshua Swift for their research collaboration. Susan Reynolds, our acquisitions editor at American Psychological Association Books, was encouraging from the start and persevering toward the end of the project; we affectionately remind her of Longfellow's observation, "Great is the art of beginning, but greater is the art of ending." We deeply appreciate our international collaborators who have faithfully translated the C-NIP into several languages (all listed on www. c-nip.net/).

Last, we mutually acknowledge each other for the pleasure of our research and writing collaboration. Working together "across the pond" proved challenging at times but nothing that persistence and technology did not overcome. We are stronger for the partnership, and we hope *Personalizing Psychotherapy* is better as well.

—John C. Norcross
Clarks Summit, PA, United States

—Mick Cooper
Brighton, United Kingdom

Personalizing Psychotherapy

1

A NEW PSYCHOTHERAPY FOR EACH PATIENT

You treat a disease, you win, you lose. You treat a person, I guarantee you'll win, no matter what the outcome.

—Patch Adams

Friday, 10:00 a.m., and Judah turns up at my (MC's) university-based clinic for an initial assessment. He is slim, pale, and tired, and he has struggled with recurring bouts of depression for about 15 years. His most recent one, triggered by feelings of envy towards a close friend, has been particularly intense: Judah has stopped working and desperately wants to rebuild his self-esteem. Judah has undergone both cognitive behavior therapy (CBT) and psychodynamic therapy before and has found the CBT focus on developing ways to cope with his anxiety—and motivating him to get out of the house—particularly helpful. He is clear that he does not want to go back into his childhood again, as he did in his psychodynamic therapy. "I really don't want to get into trying to trace the source of my problems," says Judah, "I want to focus on the present and achieving my goals."

https://doi.org/10.1037/0000221-001
Personalizing Psychotherapy: Assessing and Accommodating Patient Preferences, by J. C. Norcross and M. Cooper

At 11:30 a.m., Gabriella arrives for her appointment at my clinic, also an initial assessment. She has large dark eyes set in a rounded face and speaks in a soft Spanish accent. Like Judah, she describes the anxiety and low mood she has experienced for many years. "And would it be helpful to have goals for therapy?" I ask her. Gabriella responds, "I think it's better to leave it open. . . . Goals always put pressure on me; I feel I have to please." Gabriella explains that—at least, for the first few sessions—she would like to have an "open space" to explore her childhood, focusing on the bereavements and abandonments that she believes are at the root of her problems.

Two clients of the same age, seen at the same clinic, suffering from similar disorders, and yet there is a world of difference in terms of what they want from psychotherapy and what proves helpful for them. Nearly all mental health professionals recognize this fundamental truth: What works for one person may not work for another. The law of individual differences operates mightily in treatment outcomes. Research and experience inform the probability of generic success—80% of patients will experience improvement in psychotherapy, for instance—but not the promise of individual success. As a natural consequence, we mental health professionals seek "different strokes for different folks" (Blatt & Felsen, 1993) or to *personalize* psychotherapy.

In this opening chapter, we introduce this evidence-based, therapist-tested means of adapting psychotherapy to this essential patient characteristic. We review how the concept of personalization in psychotherapy has evolved over time, define the subject of the book (preferences), demonstrate variability across client perspectives, and canvass the rightful meaning of evidence-based practice.

HISTORY OF PERSONALIZING PSYCHOTHERAPY

Historically, the means of such matching has been to tailor the psychotherapy to the patient's diagnosis or presenting problem—that is, to find the best treatment for a particular disorder. And, indeed, the research suggests that particular treatments may prove particularly useful for a handful of disorders, such as some form of exposure for trauma and parent management training for childhood externalizing disorders (Barlow, 2014; Nathan & Gorman, 2015). However, the repeated *dodo bird* conclusion indicates that bona fide psychotherapies produce similar outcomes, once the researcher allegiance effect is identified and controlled (Wampold & Imel, 2015). The decades-long search for optimal matches between the treatment method and the patient's disorder has largely proved unsuccessful (Prochaska et al., 2020).

Nonetheless, the overwhelming majority of randomized clinical trials (RCTs) in psychotherapy still assess the efficacy of specific treatments for specific disorders. Those research studies problematically collapse numerous clients under a single diagnosis. It is a false and, to be blunt, misleading presupposition in RCTs that the patients are homogenous (Beutler & Clarkin, 1990). Perhaps the patients are diagnostically homogeneous, but nondiagnostic variability is the rule, as we saw with Judah and Gabriella. It is precisely the unique individual and the singular context that many psychotherapists attempt to treat (Norcross & Beutler, 2014).

Particularly absent from much of the controlled research and clinical training has been adapting psychotherapy to the person of the patient, beyond their disorder (Norcross & Wampold, 2019). As Sir William Osler (1906), father of modern medicine, wrote: "It is much more important to know what sort of a patient has a disease than what sort of disease a patient has." In fact, as we will see, evidence-based practice (EBP) demands that mental health professionals attend to patient characteristics, preferences, and values. But how to do so in practice constitutes the most neglected facet and the soft underbelly of EBP in mental health (Norcross et al., 2017). We are repeatedly enjoined to treat the whole person and preferences but rarely trained how to do so.

Blending patient preferences with the research evidence and clinical expertise will necessarily broaden our decision making. The traditional medical–pharmaceutical model assumes that the curative power lies primarily in the medicine or method; that is, the relationship is hierarchically structured, with the provider serving as the expert, and the patient's role is to comply and participate as prescribed (Bohart, 2005; Orlinsky, 1989). The psychosocial model, by contrast, anticipates a more comprehensive and bidirectional process. The curative power rests not only with the treatment method but also within the treatment relationship, the person of the practitioner, and the active client. Further, the therapeutic relationship works through collaboration, empathy, and support. We filter and focus all treatment decisions through the lens of the patient's characteristics, preferences, and culture. The client collaborates, remains informed, and works hard to participate and self-heal.

The psychosocial model requires us to abandon a paternalistic stance and a passive image of patients and move toward a more collaborative stance and an active image of clients. The psychosocial model, likewise, rejects monocultural, one-size-fits-all treatments for a particular diagnosis in favor of culturally informed, individually tailored care. Shared decision making is the evidence-based result.

A ROSE BY ANY OTHER NAME

The process of personalizing psychotherapy to the patient has been accorded multiple names over the years (Norcross & Wampold, 2019). In alphabetical order, 10 of these terms are

♦ aptitude by treatment interaction (a research design)
♦ attunement (referring to care carefully adjusted to patient wishes)
♦ bespoke (as in clothing made for a particular customer)
♦ customizing (also frequently used to refer to finishing an automobile)
♦ differential therapeutics (also the title of influential books, e.g., Frances et al., 1984)
♦ fitting (as in fit for a specific person)
♦ individualizing (self-explanatory nomenclature)
♦ matchmaking (also often reserved for romantic pairing by grandmothers)
♦ precision care (frequently employed in medicine)
♦ treatment selection (a more inclusive term that considers client preferences)

A series of focus groups conducted at the University of Scranton investigated laypersons' favorites among these and related terms. *Personalizing*, *individualizing*, and *tailoring* consistently emerged as the favored and intelligible terms for this process, among both actual and potential psychotherapy clients. In clinical work, we employ these three terms interchangeably because they are self-explanatory and parallel language in personalized medicine.

In professional circles, *treatment adaptation* and *responsiveness* tend to prevail. The former is generally favored by cognitive behavior therapists and the latter by relational, humanistic, and psychodynamic therapists. By whatever name, however, the goal is to enhance treatment effectiveness by tailoring it to the unique individual and their specific preferences. In other words, psychotherapists endeavor to create a new therapy for each client, in collaboration with that client.

Our overarching purposes for writing this book were presciently anticipated by George Orwell (1946/2005), who wrote about the universal motivations of all writers: "to share an experience which one feels is valuable and ought not to be missed" and "to push the world in a certain direction." That valuable experience, that future direction, is accommodating client preferences in psychotherapy.

DEFINING AND CATEGORIZING TERMS

Patient preferences in psychotherapy are defined as the specific conditions and activities that clients want in their treatment experience (Swift et al., 2019). That closely corresponds to the *Merriam Webster's Dictionary* (n.d.) definitions of *preference* as "the power or opportunity of choosing," "the act, fact, or principle of giving advantages to some over others," and "priority in the right to demand and receive satisfaction of an obligation." Preferences comprise relative or comparative rankings; sometimes, all the treatments represent disagreeable choices, and one is forced to select among "the most preferable of evils" (Homer). In this volume, the terms *favor*, *desire*, *want*, and *choose* are used synonymously with *prefer*, though the latter three terms have less of this comparative emphasis.

Our working definition refers to preferences in and about psychotherapy by the patient, which are assessed (or ignored) by the mental health professional. As we shall see, patient preferences exist and operate whether or not they are explicitly invited and considered in treatment. Our working definition excludes general life preferences of patients outside the treatment experience. It also excludes the preferences of psychotherapists: We use the terms *preferences* and *client preferences* synonymously. This is not to minimize the importance of psychotherapists' understandings and experiences— they have an essential role to play in working with client preferences, as is closely examined in this book. However, our starting point, and focus, is on what clients desire.

Most clients have hopes and desires about what will happen (preferences), in contrast to what they expect to happen (expectations). We prefer that the Philadelphia Eagles win the Super Bowl each year, or Brighton and Hove Albion win the Champions League, but we certainly do not expect it. We do not directly address client expectations in this book. They represent what clients *believe* will occur in psychotherapy, in contrast to what they *want* to occur. Certainly, these can overlap, but, for example, a Hispanic woman may strongly prefer to work with a therapist of the same ethnicity but not expect this to be available to her.

Prioritizing Strong Preferences

Strong preferences serve as the coin of this clinical realm. Our particular focus is on the assessment and accommodation of intensely held desires because they are most likely to impact treatment satisfaction and success. Had Judah (from the example at the beginning of the chapter), for instance, said that he was just a bit reluctant to talk about his past, it might not have been too problematic to make that a focus of the therapeutic work. But his statement that he really did not want to go back into it again needed close attention. In-session time is limited and valuable; we prioritize strong preferences.

When patients respond that they do not clearly favor a particular choice point, we move on to another. This is especially the case in formally assessing psychotherapy preferences. In fact, our Cooper–Norcross Inventory of Preferences (C-NIP; Chapter 5) is normed on U.S. and U.K. adults to identify strong treatment preferences (operationally defined as the highest or lowest 25% of patient responses). Keep in mind the legal maxim: *De minimis noncurat lex* ("The law does not care about trifles"). Putting a lot of clinical effort into assessing and accommodating minor preferences may distract you from incorporating more substantive matters.

Categorizing Client Preferences

Psychotherapy preferences have commonly been grouped into three categories (Swift et al., 2019). First, *treatment preferences* concern any desires that clients might have for specific types of intervention. Increasingly, patients request a specific form of treatment (e.g., psychotherapy vs. medication) or approach/orientation (e.g., cognitive behavioral, psychodynamic, humanistic). This category of preferences also covers other interventions, such as bibliotherapy or support groups (e.g., McLeod, 2012; Norcross et al., 2013; Tompkins et al., 2017).

Second, *preferences about the therapist* concern the type of practitioner with whom clients would like to work. These inclinations are often based on the practitioners' sociodemographic characteristics, such as gender, ethnicity, and age, although research has indicated that clients frequently report even stronger preferences for a therapist's interpersonal and personality characteristics (Swift et al., 2015).

Third, *activity preferences* refer to the specific actions that clients desire to engage in throughout the psychotherapy process. This is a more micro-level focus than treatment preferences, the latter referring to the overall package of activities that the client desires. Activity preferences can be in such areas as therapeutic methods (e.g., two-chair work, behavioral experiments), the therapist's style of engagement (e.g., friendly, challenging), or understandings of the client's problems (e.g., biological, behavioral). Activity preferences also include the particular format of psychotherapy that the client wants. For instance, some clients enter psychotherapy specifically requesting couple sessions, whereas others insist on individual work. After the COVID-19 pandemic, some clients continue to prefer telehealth instead of in-person sessions.

The distinction between treatment preferences and activity preferences tends, admittedly, to blur, but the goal is to attend to both types. One of us (JCN) spends proportionally more time assessing the macro-level treatment preferences toward the beginning of therapy; that, as you will see, has the benefit of more research support because the vast majority of empirical investigations have been conducted on those. The other (MC) spends relatively more time gauging the micro-level activity preferences for particular sessions; that, as you will read, has the advantage of responding flexibly to the flow of client needs. Strike the difference between us and honor both strong treatment and activity desires.

Each of the three preference types is critical at the point of initial assessment, but treatment and therapist preferences tend to recede in importance once the actual course of psychotherapy has commenced (unless clients want to change their psychotherapist or their intervention package). Activity preferences, however, stay relevant throughout the therapeutic processes and may be assessed, examined, and adjusted on a regular—even session-by-session—basis. In this respect, we can distinguish between *between-treatment preferences*, which shape the particular course of psychotherapy, and *within-treatment preferences*, which influence the course of psychotherapy once that treatment has commenced.

Preferences for therapist demographics and competencies probably play the largest role in decisions about starting therapy. For two examples, a client with limited English fluency prefers a Spanish-speaking therapist, and another patient might desire only psychoactive medication. However, once therapy begins, the practitioner's in-session style and behaviors take the front stage.

We can also distinguish between several elements of preference work. *Preference assessment* refers to the identification of the client's wants for psychotherapy. This is similar to *preference elicitation*—bringing those wants to the fore—but the process of preference assessment implies that the psychotherapist plays a more active role in interpreting those wants. Then we have *preference accommodation*, where the counselor adjusts their way of working to the client's expressed wants and desires. This is likely to lead to *preference matching*, where the client receives the particular treatment, activity, or type of therapist that they indicate. Note, though, that preference matching can occur without preference accommodation: There is always the possibility that what is offered and what is desired will spontaneously coincide. Finally, there is *preference discussion* when psychotherapist and patient talk together about what it is that the patient wants and how that can best be accommodated.

Shared Decision Making

A concept closely related to preference assessment and accommodation, with its roots in the medical field, is *shared decision making* (SDM). This is commonly defined as

> a process in which clinicians and patients work together to select tests, treatments, management, or support packages, based on clinical evidence and patients' informed preferences. It involves the provision of evidence-based information about options, outcomes and uncertainties, together with decision support counselling and systems for recording and implementing patients' treatment preferences. (Coulter & Collins, 2011, p. vii)

In contrast to preference assessment and accommodation, the focus of SDM is most commonly on specific, one-off treatment decisions, such as whether or not to have surgery for prostate cancer, rather than also including ongoing, within-treatment assessments and adjustments. Nevertheless, as applied in psychotherapy practice and certainly in terms of its ethics and values, SDM can be considered synonymous with client preference work. For this reason, we discuss the evidence base for SDM alongside the research evidence for preference assessment and accommodation in the following chapter.

SDM is indeed shared. It rejects the traditional, *paternalistic* model of health care, in which the practitioner decides what is best, but it also rejects the *informed choice* model, in which the patient is simply given information and left to make the decision by themselves (Makoul & Clayman, 2006). In other words, SDM, as with preference assessment and accommodation in psychotherapy, emphasizes a "midpoint" of dialogue and communication, with both psychotherapist and patient playing an active part.

This SDM continuum can be nuanced further into shared but more psychotherapist led, shared equally, and shared but more client led (Gibson et al., 2020). Hence, decision making in psychotherapy exists on a 5-point spectrum (see Figure 1.1), ranging from wholly paternalistic, therapist-led decisions to those that are wholly client led, with SDM covering a range of collaborative possibilities in between.

WHAT PATIENTS PREFER DIFFERS MIGHTILY

Clinicians need to select the best treatment for the particular contextualized individual sitting in front of them, not the treatment that purportedly works best for the hypothetical average patient. Averaging flattens and devalues individual experience; research evidence is derived from groups of people, yet we make decisions for and with individuals. Treatment effects are

FIGURE 1.1. The Spectrum of Shared Decision Making

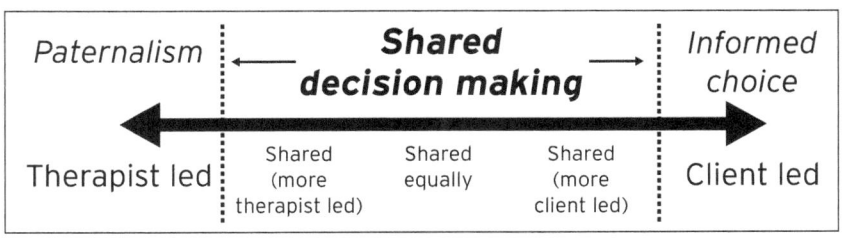

Note. Data from Gibson et al. (2020).

invariably heterogeneous (Kent et al., 2019); it is the essential individual differences at the core of psychological therapy. The consequences are obvious but monumental. We improve the efficacy of mental health care by individualizing care.

Virtually all our patients desire relief from suffering but vary widely in how to achieve it. This is Psychology 101: the law of individual differences, client heterogeneity, individual variability, our undeniable uniqueness.

Try asking friends, colleagues, students, and patients what they would strongly prefer in their psychotherapy or psychotherapist. Prepare to marvel at the huge variations in their answers. Some clamor for weekly homework, others despise such assignments; some want constant support and emotional hugs, others seek professional detachment and objective analysis. Some specifically seek dialectical behavior therapy, and others seek psychoanalytic therapy. A prominent humanistic practitioner once surprised me (JCN) by saying that he wanted "someone who would challenge and push me." The quizzical look on my face, communicating a "but you are a person-centered, low-directive therapist," was immediately met with, "You asked what I wanted for myself, not what I give to my patients."

Research consistently underscores the wide variation in what clients favor in psychological care. Consider patient responses to a few (of the 18) C-NIP items. On each item, clients select an answer to "I would like the therapist to . . ." on a 7-point scale with 3, 2, and 1 indicating strong, moderate, and slight preferences, respectively, in the chosen direction (and 0 indicating no or equal preferences). Figure 1.2 presents responses from over 1,300 laypeople to items assessing temporal focus, and Figure 1.3 presents their preferences regarding the amount of treatment structure.

Clients favor positions across the entire spectrum of preferences. Some desire an exclusive focus on their future, others a past orientation, and most a combination of the two. Some clients strongly desire that the therapy be

FIGURE 1.2. U.S. and U.K. Laypeople Preferences for Temporal Focus

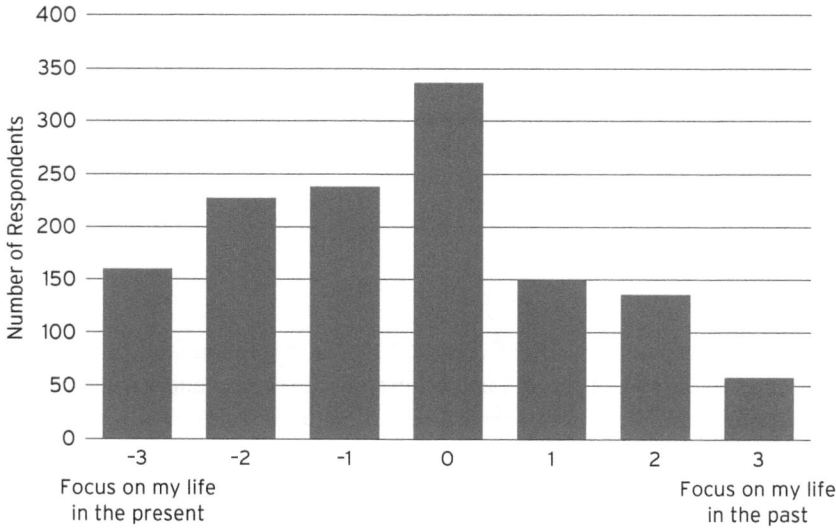

Note. Data from Cooper et al. (2017).

FIGURE 1.3. U.S. and U.K. Laypeople Preferences for Structured and Unstructured Therapy

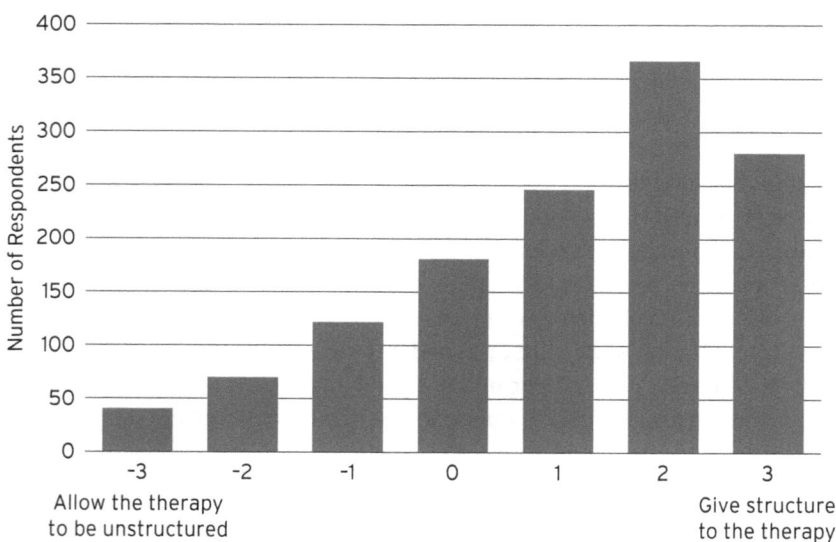

Note. Data from Cooper, Norcross, et al. (2019).

unstructured, whereas more clients strongly request that the practitioner give structure to the therapy. Similar response patterns are evident in the other C-NIP items as well: Patient variability rules.

WHAT PATIENTS WANT AND WHAT PATIENTS GET

Currently, in health care systems around the world, there are substantial disparities between the kinds of treatments that patients want and the kinds of treatments that they actually receive. In one of the largest studies focusing on this question, more than 5,000 people from the general public in Germany completed a structured face-to-face interview about mental health treatments (Riedel-Heller et al., 2005). Interviewees were provided a vignette depicting someone who was experiencing depression and one for schizophrenia. They were then asked to rank order their preferred treatments among five options (psychotherapy, medication, natural remedies, relaxation, and meditation/yoga). For depression, more than half preferred psychotherapy, 18% preferred relaxation, 12% preferred natural remedies, and only 11% preferred medication. For schizophrenia, almost two thirds preferred psychotherapy, and only 15% preferred medication. In actuality, more than half of people suffering from those two disorders receive only medication. The prevalence of treatments, however, displays convincingly that consumer voices are largely ignored and that people do not routinely receive what they desire.

Another stark illustration of how patients rarely receive their treatment preferences hails from 411 parents of adolescents receiving psychological treatment (Becker et al., 2018). Here, 43% of parents preferred to receive a therapist referral from their pediatrician, 30% from another parent, and few from an insurance company. But 27% actually received the referral from an insurance company, and only 15% received the recommendation from a fellow parent. The majority of parents (53%) wanted their adolescent to receive therapy from a center focused on adolescents, but only 16% actually did so. The disconnect between desire and reality is manifest in mental health care. It frequently represents a variant of the Rolling Stones famous refrain: You can't always get what you want, and sometimes you don't even get what you need.

OUR PATH TO PREFERENCE RESEARCH

We have each been assessing and researching psychotherapy preferences for about 10 to 15 years now. This pursuit came naturally to us as integrative or pluralistic psychologists striving to flexibly attune treatment to the unique individual and the singular situation. But several memorable clients pushed us to privilege how our clients desired to work in session.

For one of us (JCN), two patients in particular permanently raised my clinical antenna. The first, let's call her "Danielle," was a middle-aged Hispanic woman referred to me by her internist for exposure therapy following two episodes of unsuccessful treatment (medication monotherapy by a psychiatrist and generic counseling by a social worker). Danielle was suffering from severe posttraumatic stress disorder (PTSD) and moderate depression, now becoming chronic (2 years and counting). Toward the end of our initial meeting, I asked Danielle whether she had any strong preferences for her psychotherapy. She tentatively suggested in a soft voice that perhaps the space between us was "too open, too intense; maybe something could be put between us?" (My default office configuration is two chairs facing each other, at a slight angle.) I reflected that her preference seemed right, and natural, for someone feeling vulnerable and struggling with interpersonal trauma. She smiled as I stood and moved a small coffee table between us and moved my chair a foot further away from hers. I would do so for the next eight sessions when she appeared for weekly appointments. At the eighth session, she entered the office and observed that the furniture restructuring was no longer necessary; "It's fine just as it is," she said. By the 10th session, Danielle was terminating after a successful course of EMDR (eye-movement desensitization and reprocessing). As is my wont, I inquired in our termination sessions about what worked and what did not in our contacts. She immediately replied—and her response is imprinted on my brain—"That's easy: You asked what I wanted and then tried to accomplish it. That's when I knew you cared and that psychotherapy would work this time."

The second memorable case for me (JCN), "Diane," had been dumped, unceremoniously and unexpectedly, by her longtime boyfriend in the middle of her senior year in high school (Prochaska & Norcross, 2018). And the boyfriend left Diane for a good friend of hers! She said her heart felt like it had been ripped out and thrown on the floor. She exhibited an adjustment reaction with mixed emotional features, alternating between grief and rage, one moment sobbing and unable to get out of bed, the next moment fantasizing some murderous payback. He was her first true love, her first sexual partner, and her first soul mate. To complicate matters, Diane's mother seemed as upset as she was. Her mother offered support and comfort; after all, she was a talented psychodynamic psychiatrist who hinted darkly to Diane at home and to me in the referral call of "relational vulnerabilities" and "emotional traumatization" resulting from this breakup. The mother/ therapist was expecting many months, perhaps years, of weekly intensive psychotherapy to address the roots of the problem. But Diane expressed the opposite treatment preferences: She wanted to dig out of her crisis, not dig into the archaeology of her emotional life. When I asked her to identify her treatment goals and preferences, she instantly replied, "Not to let this jerk spoil the rest of my senior year. To get back my life. And to do it quickly." Diane knew the path to her health and how to proceed. Despite her mother's preferences for months of uncovering psychotherapy, Diane realized her goals in just four sessions (plus an intake session). She called on her considerable skills and resources as a college-bound student to develop a plan to get her life back. Diane consumed the best-seller *Reviving Ophelia* (Pipher, 1994) in one night, declaring that she too had totally lost her self in a romantic relationship, like many adolescent women. At the close of our final session, just 2 months after we initially met, Diane turned to me and said, "We've really surprised Mom. She was pissed at first that we decided to only meet every two weeks. If she had her way, you would have seen me twice a week. But as much as I love her, sometimes the patient knows what's best for her, not the therapist" (Prochaska & Norcross, 2018).

My (MC's) journey to appreciating and prioritizing client preferences was more of a gradual transition. I was trained as a pure existential psychotherapist, focusing on clients' phenomenological experiences and working in a strictly descriptive way (Cooper, 2015, 2017). I then went on to teach and research in the person-centered field: again, a relatively descriptive form of practicing (Cooper et al., 2010, 2013). I loved the client-centered, relational values of both these approaches—putting the patient's subjective experiences at the heart of the therapy—but came to realize that these practices, themselves, could be quite inflexible and (paradoxically) therapist centered. When I came out of training, I was—and I hate to admit this—too rigid, too definite, and too one-size-fits-all. I remember sitting opposite clients in blank, silent spaces, thinking, "What are we actually doing here?" It did not seem to be what clients wanted, and I did not know where we were going. Most important, perhaps, I sometimes felt a coldness and distance between us. We were on different pages: me with my existential and person-centered theories of what might help the client and the client with quite different understandings of what they wanted and needed.

Over time, the shackles of my training and my own desire for certainty began to loosen. I started to see the value of different ways of practicing. And when I began to ask my clients how they wanted to work, a whole new world of possibilities opened. Now I was relating, not on my own phenomenological terms, but in a much more human, flexible, and interactive way. I was back in myself. This was, I recognized, what it meant to be client centered: opening myself up to the client's own ideas about growth and genuinely respecting their perspective. I was practicing more effectively with each of my clients, making the most of our unique interactions. My practice felt more creative, more responsive, and more effective. More than all of that, though, the difference was that I was genuinely meeting each of my clients: engaging with them as one flawed human being to another.

I started to write with one of my colleagues, John McLeod, about this way of working, which we called *pluralistic* (Cooper & McLeod, 2007, 2011): therapy that is personalized to the unique wants and needs of each client. "Pluralism" can be considered synonymous with "integration" but with a particular emphasis on personalization and client–therapist collaboration. It also links integrative thinking and practice back to a tradition of progressive, democratic philosophy, such as the work of William James (1909/1996) and Isaiah Berlin (1958).

PREFERENCES ARE NOT THE ONLY THING

Patient preferences and values related to treatment are a primary, but not the sole, consideration in forming a therapeutic relationship and selecting methods. Other prominent factors include

- variations in presenting problems, etiology, and comorbid syndromes
- chronological age, developmental status, and developmental history
- sociocultural factors, including gender, gender identity, ethnicity, race, social class, religion, disability status, and sexual orientation
- environmental context (e.g., institutional racism, health-care disparities) and stressors (e.g., unemployment, major life events)
- readiness to change
- treatment acceptability
- availability
- probability of payer approval
- caregiver agreement
- prior treatment failures
- intolerable side effects

Take the case of Francesco, a quiet, polite 30-year-old Hispanic man who presented at a low-income primary health-care center with generalized anxiety and an extensive history of alcohol dependence (Norcross et al., 2017). His marriage had recently ended in a divorce, and his $12 per hour factory job was in jeopardy due to layoffs and outsourcing. His job did not provide health insurance, and as a single working man, Francesco did not qualify for any heavily discounted state- or federally-funded insurance. Here, Francesco's strong preferences for an inpatient alcohol rehabilitation followed by weekly outpatient therapy paled in comparison to his dire economic considerations. Any shared decision making that does not account for the patient's socioeconomic context is ripe for failure.

The explicit enumeration and delicate balancing of these multiple patient considerations bring the underlying value judgments into bold relief (Guyatt et al., 2008). Whose values—practitioners, patients, insurers, society—do we see reflected in treatment decisions? And do we find those values (and their sources) explicitly articulated?

URGENT QUESTIONS AND IMMEDIATE ANSWERS

At this point, during our clinical workshops and professional presentations on psychotherapy preferences, a concern often surfaces about "willy-nilly giving patients whatever they want!" Let us address here such recurrent, pressing questions, to which we respond in greater depth and with more precision in later chapters.

So, just give clients whatever they desire?!

Of course not. Legal, ethical, and clinical considerations constantly operate as well, and none of us can offer all 450-plus forms of psychotherapy out there. But we invariably invite patients to talk about their preferences, and doing so when we cannot accommodate them is as important as when we can.

Most clients don't know what they want, so why ask?

It's certainly true that some clients don't have strong preferences—particularly if they haven't been in psychotherapy before—but research shows that most do (see Chapter 3). It's also about how a clinician asks: A patient may not have many answers to the direct question "What do you want from psychotherapy?" but more subtle and exploratory questions—such as "What would be helpful here?" "What's useful to you when you're struggling?" or "What do you especially dislike in counseling?"—may produce fuller responses.

Isn't it the therapist's responsibility to select the treatment plan?

Yes and no. Yes, the mental health professional possesses the training and expertise to recommend a treatment. No, the mental health professional does not unilaterally impose a treatment except in the most urgent situations. The days of psychotherapist paternalism are gone; all ethical codes dictate collaborative decision making with clients.

Doesn't this already occur routinely in good health care?

In theory, yes; in reality, probably not. Research shows that health care professionals think they are doing more shared decision making than their patients report. Try this thought experiment: Think of the last three times you consulted a health care professional. How many times were you asked about an important treatment preference? Not many times with us either. The sole exception (in the United States) is "How do you prefer to pay the bill?"

But surely psychotherapists are better than that, right?

Probably so. At the same time, having watched and listened to thousands of hours of session recordings, we see little evidence that mental health professionals regularly or explicitly assess patient preferences or engage in extended discussions about them. Therapists often assess the patient's goals for psychotherapy (the destination; where to go) but rarely the patient's preferences about psychotherapy (the journey; how to get there). Our research colleagues Joshua Swift and Roger Greenberg (2015) flatly declared, "Although most therapists would say that they care about their clients' opinions and desires for treatment, actually taking steps to accommodate client preferences doesn't often occur" (p. 79).

A study on how mental health professionals choose among several treatments for PTSD bears this out (Simiola et al., 2019). Clinicians identified their multiple selection considerations: 78% said their belief in the treatment's efficacy, 37% their own preferences, 25% integrating treatment approaches, 27% type and nature of the index trauma, 45% symptom presentation, 40% patient's cognitive style, 17% patient's treatment history, and 23% patient's preferences. Only 23% based treatment selection on the client's preference! It bears reminding that client preference is, by far, the best research-supported and most effective way from the preceding criteria for choosing among treatment methods, but less than a quarter of these highly trained professionals did so.

Fair enough, but how do you suggest we evaluate those preferences, especially as we do not have a lot of session time to do so?

We experienced the same clinical predicament, and that's why we constructed the brief and multidimensional C-NIP.

(Audible sigh). Another measure to purchase, another measure to administer and score, another piece of paper . . .

Nope. The C-NIP is a free measure in the public domain (www.c-nip.net/). The C-NIP averages 3 minutes to administer and self-score, and clients generally find it a valuable addition to psychotherapy. They can also take it online if they like.

Well, what happens if I cannot meet the patient's preferences after I assess them?

Three things probably ensue. First, the client is grateful and impressed that you asked what they desired. The research demonstrates that you strengthen the therapeutic alliance and decrease treatment dropout simply by assessing preferences. Second, you initiate a respectful dialogue in which you discuss your reasons for not offering the preferred services and elicit the patient's honest reactions. And third, you collaborate with the client in determining the next treatment steps, whether that be an adapted version of what they want, an alternative to what they want, or the suggestion of another service or professional.

And if I can accommodate the patient's strong preferences?

Then you and your patient typically reap the benefits: reduced treatment dropout, stronger therapy relationship, and improved psychotherapy outcome. Plus, you comply with your profession's ethical code and render evidence-based care.

So, join with us, friend, as we unpack the research-supported and practice-tested virtues of assessing and accommodating patient preferences in the following chapters.

2 THE RESEARCH EVIDENCE

The mark of a civilized human being is the ability to read a column of numbers and weep.

—Bertrand Russell

A wide variety of treatment preferences can and have been studied in the empirical research. Researchers have compared client choices among different approaches/orientations (e.g., cognitive behavioral, psychodynamic, experiential), formats of psychotherapy (e.g., group, family, individual), lengths of psychotherapy, and characteristics of psychotherapists (e.g., genders, ethnicities, sexual orientations, personality characteristics). They have also asked clients to express preferences for psychotherapy versus medication versus combined treatment, self-help versus formal treatment, and in-person care versus internet-based health care.

This large and growing research base has canvassed a multitude of behavioral disorders among virtually all client populations. Recent studies have addressed client preferences in anxiety conditions, alcohol misuse,

https://doi.org/10.1037/0000221-002
Personalizing Psychotherapy: Assessing and Accommodating Patient Preferences, by J. C. Norcross and M. Cooper

obesity, and much more. The clinical populations have consisted of children, adolescents, adults, and older adults across the multitude of treatment settings. And across these diverse disorders, clients, treatments, and populations, the research has been consistently enthusiastic (at least as enthusiastic as research can be): Accommodating patient preferences works!

In this chapter, we provide a practice-friendly review of this research evidence. Our aim is to be, at once, scholarly and practical, reducing what James Joyce characterized as "the true scholastic stink" to bearable levels. We focus primarily on the *meta-analyses* (studies of studies) that summarize the preference research and highlight the central findings and clinical implications.

REPRESENTATIVE STUDIES

Let's begin by describing representative studies that populate the preference literature and serve as the primary data for the meta-analyses. Prospective patients with mental health diagnoses are recruited for a research study and are administered a variety of psychopathology and personality measures, at least one of which assesses a preference for psychotherapy (e.g., talking therapy or medication, cognitive behavior therapy [CBT] or psychodynamic therapy, female or male therapist). In the strongest type of study design, patients are then randomly assigned to receive either their preferred approach (matched) or something other than their preferences (mismatched or unmatched). Alternatively, rather than being matched to their preferences, in some study designs, patients may be allocated to a treatment-as-usual (TAU) condition in which they simply receive a treatment irrespective of their preferences.

Say a patient explicitly favors CBT during the intake assessment. If the patient is randomly assigned to her preference, then she receives the desired intervention (match). If, however, the patient is randomly assigned to not her preference, then she receives person-centered psychotherapy (mismatch or unmatched), for example. But if the design involves random assignment to TAU, the patient may be allocated to whichever treatment might be available next, which may or may not be CBT.

Probably the earliest study of preference effects to be included in the meta-analyses was conducted by Devine and Fernald (1973). They investigated the potential impact of receiving preferred, nonpreferred, or randomly allocated group treatments for snake phobia (Swift et al., 2019). The researchers randomized clients to match/choice and mismatch/no-choice conditions. The study involved 48 participants with an extreme fear of snakes: 32 of them were shown a 40-minute video that described and illustrated four approaches to treating snake phobia. The treatments were systematic desensitization, an "encounter approach" (which explored personal feelings), rational emotive therapy focusing on irrational thoughts, and a modeling or behavioral rehearsal approach. Thirty-two participants then expressed their liking for each approach on a 5-point scale and were assigned to a treatment for which they either expressed a strong liking or disliking. The remaining 16 participants, who did not watch the video, were randomly allocated to one of the four treatments. Hence, 12 clients participated in each treatment: four who expressed a liking for it, four who expressed a dislike for it, and four who were randomly allocated to it. Each therapy lasted for two 1-hour sessions. At follow-up, the 16 participants who had received their preferred treatment showed significantly less fear of snakes than their counterparts who received a nonpreferred therapy or had been randomly assigned.

A larger scale study of the preference effect hails from the classic National Institute of Mental Health Treatment of Depression Collaborative Research Program. This analyzed the relation between patients' beliefs about their treatments and their treatment engagement and outcomes (Elkin et al., 1999). The researchers did not assign patients to their preferences, but rather analyzed data from clients randomized to different treatments. This multisite trial compared the effectiveness of (a) CBT, (b) interpersonal psychotherapy (IPT), (c) antidepressant with clinical management, and (d) placebo with clinical management across 250 clients suffering from major depressive disorder.

Patients' preferences for treatment were inferred based on their predilections for each treatment. This was patients' "beliefs about the origins of their distress and their expectations about what will be helpful to them" (Elkin et al., 1999, p. 438). On the basis of responses to several items from a predilection questionnaire, patients were classified as having a preference for a particular treatment if they scored above the midpoint on the scale that corresponded to that treatment and if this score was at least one point higher than their scores for the two other scales. This resulted in 43 patients with a CBT preference, four for IPT, and 24 for medication. In addition, the researchers identified 28 patients as having a preference for psychotherapy of either type.

Elkin and colleagues (1999) compared engagement outcomes for patients who received a treatment congruent with their predilections with those who received a treatment that was noncongruent with their predilections. The four measures of engagement were early dropout; patients' ratings of their therapists' empathy, warmth, and genuineness; observers' ratings of the clients' contribution to the therapeutic alliance; and depressive symptoms. The analyses indicated that patients receiving their preferred treatment were significantly less likely to drop out prematurely. The differences in dropout between congruent/match and noncongruent/unmatched groups were dramatic: 5% versus 21%, respectively. Moreover, two thirds of the patients who dropped out directly indicated that a major determinant had been dissatisfaction with treatment or desire for another treatment. In addition, patients in the congruent/preference match group had significantly higher ratings of the therapist-provided therapeutic conditions and significantly higher ratings on the patient's contribution to the therapeutic alliance (Swift et al., 2019).

Not all studies show a preference effect. For instance, Kerns and associates (2014) looked at whether a tailored CBT intervention for chronic back pain—which incorporated clients' preferences for particular therapeutic skills and strategies—would improve treatment engagement and participation compared with standard CBT. They found no differences between the groups in the numbers of dropouts or sessions attended. The study was well-powered, with over 60 participants in each group, but, of course, it was just one study in one area focusing on a particular form of preference accommodation. The great advantage of meta-analyses, then, is that they can aggregate multiple findings from multiple studies to give an overall indication of effects.

PREFERENCE MEASURES IN THE RESEARCH

Before looking at the results of the meta-analyses, let us consider how preferences are measured, as the method and context of assessing patient preferences probably influence their eventual choices. Some studies present the choices via interview, audiotape, videotape, or written forms. Context may be responsible for some of the inconsistent results across studies and investigators. Bear that caution in mind as you traverse this chapter.

Consider an early study (Coursol & Sipps, 1986) that tried to reconcile the conflicting literature: Some studies reported a general preference for behavioral therapies, whereas other studies found a preference for insight-oriented therapies. More than 300 college students rated their preferences for both theoretical orientations. The behavioral orientation received a significantly higher preference when presented audiovisually as a therapy session, but the person-centered orientation received the higher preference when presented as a written description. Which, then, was favored? It depends on the measure and context.

Probably the most popular measure in research has been to directly ask patients which approach they would prefer to receive—for instance, asking whether they prefer medication or psychotherapy or whether they prefer a male or female therapist (Swift et al., 2019). In a variation of this direct self-report, some studies provided patients with descriptions and/or demonstrations of several approaches prior to asking them to state a preference.

In contrast, some researchers have employed questionnaires or rating scales that assess preference strength as well as preferences, per se. Assessing preference strength is of value because one might expect that stronger preferences, compared with weaker preferences, would exert greater influence on treatment outcomes. For example, researchers have not only invited depressed patients to indicate whether they preferred psychotherapy or pharmacotherapy but also asked them to rate on a 5-point, Likert-type scale how strongly they wanted their preferred treatment. (We review the formal preference measures in Chapter 5.)

In research settings, investigators have occasionally employed *delay-discounting methods* to assess the strength of psychotherapy preferences. Traditionally used in economics, this method measures individuals' preferences for smaller immediate rewards compared with larger delayed ones. Individuals are asked, for instance, whether they prefer to receive $10 today or $20 in 1 week. Depending on the initial choice, the delayed reward can be raised or lowered to find the value that individuals place on time over money.

In a pioneering study, Swift and Callahan (2010) asked 57 adult clients how much they were willing to sacrifice in terms of treatment efficacy to receive a therapist with whom they could develop a positive working relationship. Clients were initially asked whether they would prefer a treatment that had been found to work for about 70% of clients in recent clinical trials but was delivered by a therapist who was difficult to relate to, or a treatment that had been found to work for about 10% of clients in recent clinical trials but was delivered by a therapist who was easy for them to relate to. Although most clients initially picked the 70% option, on average, they switched to the less effective treatment once it reached 30%—thus indicating they were willing to sacrifice 40% in treatment efficacy to ensure that positive therapeutic relationship.

Swift and colleagues (2015) used the same method with preferences for racial/ethnic therapists. They determined that participants had much stronger preferences for therapist multicultural training and use of culturally adapted treatments than they did for simple racial/ethnic matching with therapists.

Using a similar delay-discounting method, Boswell and colleagues (2018) asked 403 community mental health patients to determine the relative value of clinician performance information. Overall, and not surprisingly, patients valued learning about the track record of practitioners' effectiveness. But they also preferred practitioners who charged less and with whom there was a high likelihood of establishing a good alliance. The patients, as a group, preferred more effective, less expensive, and high alliance psychotherapists to about the same degree. Lower in strength were such preferences as same-ethnicity or same-gender therapist.

META-ANALYTIC REVIEWS ON PREFERENCES

Several meta-analyses have examined the effect of patient preferences on mental health outcomes (Lindhiem et al., 2014; Preference Collaborative Review Group & McPherson, 2009; Swift et al., 2011, 2019; Windle et al., 2019). The meta-analyses included overlapping studies and generally reached similar conclusions: receiving the favored treatment results in lower dropout rates and better clinical outcomes. Hence, here we summarize the two largest and most recent meta-analyses.

Effect of Preference Accommodation on Treatment Outcomes

Swift and colleagues (2019) sought to include all studies published in the English language that quantitatively examined the impact of preference accommodation on treatment dropout or other treatment outcomes. To be included, studies had to either assess preferences directly and then compare preference match and nonmatch conditions or include a comparison of conditions where clients were placed into choice or no-choice conditions. The researchers excluded studies of family therapy, couples therapy, and treatments for children and adolescents. This decision was made because it is more difficult to determine whose preferences informed decisions that impact dropout and outcomes (e.g., a child client whose preferences are not matched may still complete treatment if his or her parents' preferences are met; in couples therapy, one partner's preferences may be matched, whereas the other's preferences are not matched). Clinical outcomes could be a measure of the therapeutic alliance, client satisfaction, or treatment outcome (e.g., behavioral or symptom measures, frequency of heavy drinking). Fifty-three studies met their inclusion criteria and were included in this meta-analysis.

Two effect sizes were calculated for each outcome measure. First, an odds ratio (*OR*) represented the likelihood of a mismatched/no-choice client dropping out over a matched/choice client dropping out. An *OR* greater than 1 indicated that mismatched/no-choice clients were more likely to drop out prematurely, an *OR* less than 1 indicated that matched/choice clients were more likely to drop out prematurely, and an *OR* of 1 indicated that clients in both groups were equally likely to drop out. Second, Cohen's *d* represented differences in the degree of improvement between matched/choice and mismatched/no-choice groups. Table 2.1 presents several practical ways to interpret the effect size of *d* or *g*.

Regarding dropout, analysis of data from 28 studies (3,237 clients) revealed that the overall preference effect for treatment completion was

TABLE 2.1. Practical Interpretation of *d* or *g* Values

d or *g*	Cohen's benchmark	Type of effect	Percentile of treated patients[a]	Success rate of treated patients[b]
1.00		Beneficial	84	72%
.90		Beneficial	82	70%
.80	Large	Beneficial	79	69%
.70		Beneficial	76	66%
.60		Beneficial	73	64%
.50	Medium	Beneficial	69	62%
.40		Beneficial	66	60%
.30		Beneficial	62	57%
.20	Small	Beneficial	58	55%
.10		No effect	54	52%
.00		No effect	50	50%
−.10		No effect	46	48%
−.20		Detrimental	42	45%
−.30		Detrimental	38	43%

Note. Adapted from *Statistical Power Analysis for the Behavioral Sciences* (2nd ed.), by J. Cohen, 1988, Erlbaum. Copyright 1988 by Erlbaum. Also adapted from *Psychotherapy Relationships That Work: Volume 2. Evidence-Based Responsiveness* (3rd ed.), by J. C. Norcross and B. E. Wampold (Eds.), 2019, Oxford University Press. Copyright 2019 by Oxford University Press.
[a]Each effect size can be conceptualized as reflecting a corresponding percentile value; in this case, the percentile standing of the average treated patient after psychotherapy relative to untreated patients.
[b]Each effect size can also be translated into a success rate of treated patients relative to untreated patients; a *d* of .80, for example, would translate into approximately 70% of patients being treated successfully compared with 50% of untreated patients.

highly significant, both statistically and clinically. The *OR* of 1.79 (95% CI [1.44, 2.22]) indicated that clients whose preferences were not matched or who were not given a choice of their treatment conditions were 1.79 times more likely to terminate prematurely than clients who were matched to their preference or who were given a choice of their conditions. That's a huge impact: Patients not assigned to their preferred treatment were almost twice as likely to leave treatment early!

These findings are consistent with those from a separate meta-analysis of 31 randomized controlled trials looking at interventions that can substantially increase attendance at psychotherapy sessions (Oldham et al., 2012). The single most effective method is to give patients a choice of appointment time or therapist. (Preparation for psychotherapy, informational interventions, and attendance reminders also proved effective.)

Regarding psychotherapy outcome, Swift et al.'s (2019) analysis of data from 51 studies (16,269 clients) also found a highly significant effect of preference accommodation ($d = 0.28$). This effect size indicated a small to moderate meaningful difference in outcomes in favor of clients given their preferred psychotherapy. Calculation of the "fail-safe *N*" indicated that 4,177 unpublished studies with nonsignificant results would be necessary to reduce the outcome effect size to a nonsignificant level.

These meta-analytic results are both precise (based on the confidence intervals) and robust (calculation of the fail-safe *N*). Nonetheless, the results are influenced by several moderators. For example, significant differences in the preference outcome effect were found between study designs. Namely, a higher preference outcome effect was found in studies that randomized clients according to treatment conditions ($d = 0.36$), as opposed to studies that did not randomize. Thus, in research and in practice, we can expect even better outcomes when all clients are assigned to their favored care. Preference effects also depended on the outcome measure. It was highest for the therapeutic alliance and relationship variables ($d = 0.51$) and practically 0 for client satisfaction ($d = 0.03$). For actual treatment outcomes, the preference effect was in between ($d = 0.23$). Preference effects were not found to vary significantly by preference type (treatment vs. therapist vs. activity preferences).

Preference accommodation may have a larger or smaller effect depending on the client; however, patient age, gender, and years of education did not manifest any group differences in the meta-analyses. That is to say, the impact of preference was similar across populations. The size of the preference effect among patients of color is still unknown because too few studies have been conducted to compare the power of the effect to White patients, but it is at least as large. In terms of problem type, the largest preference effects were observed in treatments for anxiety, while clients with substance use disorders seemed to show lower effects. Further examination of the psychotherapy preference effect has also indicated that the preference matching effect may be particularly important in briefer interventions (Swift et al., 2013). That is, the shorter the contact, the more effective it is to accommodate the clients' likes (and dislikes).

Windle and colleagues (2019) independently assessed the effect of patient treatment preference on dropout rates and treatment outcomes. As with Swift et al. (2019), the analyses were restricted to adults, psychosocial interventions, and patients with mental health diagnoses. Multiple patient outcomes were examined: attendance, dropout, alliance, satisfaction, and symptom reduction. The meta-analysis included 29 studies, comprising 5,294 patients.

Receiving a preferred mental health treatment exerted a medium reduction in dropout risk (relative risk = 0.62) and a positive impact on the therapeutic alliance ($d = 0.48$). Both findings replicate those of Swift et al. (2019) in a smaller but overlapping set of studies. Windle and colleagues (2019) found no evidence of a significant association with outcome, but they partitioned those small number of studies into separate categories, unlike Swift et al. Overall, then, these meta-analytic findings essentially replicate the earlier meta-analyses that accommodating client preferences in mental health treatment decreases dropouts and increases the alliance and probably outcome (depending on how it is measured and aggregated).

Even Larger Effects?

These reported meta-analytic effect sizes may systematically underestimate the actual impact of accommodating patient preferences in at least two ways. First, the meta-analyses include data from all patients, even those not expressing a strong inclination. If a patient were 60–40 on one therapy over another or favored medication over psychotherapy by the thinnest of margins at 51–49, then that patient and preference was still included in the study. In clinical practice, by contrast, practitioners naturally assess and follow up on what matters—strong preferences. When research studies begin to analyze outcome differences among patients with strong preferences on treatment decisions that matter to them (not to researchers), it may well be that the emerging effect sizes will be larger. Second, as we have seen, some studies in the meta-analyses matched patients to TAU, and some of those TAU patients actually received preferred treatment.

Preference for Psychological Versus Pharmacological Treatment

Meta-analytic research has also been conducted on a frequent treatment preference: medication and/or psychotherapy. A meta-analysis of 34 English-language studies estimated the proportion of patients preferring psychological treatment relative to medication for mental disorders (McHugh et al., 2013). Seventy-five percent of adults preferred psychotherapy across the studies; this was consistently the case for both treatment-seeking and -nonseeking populations. Younger patients and women were significantly even more likely to choose psychological treatment. Clients are 3 times more likely to want psychotherapy than psychotropic drugs.

At the same time, there has been a steady decline in the percentages of patients receiving psychotherapy, along with a concomitant increase in the use of psychotropic medication. The disconnect is profound: Scores of controlled trials have demonstrated that psychotherapy is as effective as medications for a host of mental disorders, and the vast majority of patients prefer psychotherapy, yet medications alone continue to proliferate.

The tenets of evidence-based practice dictate that, without reliable evidence for the superiority of one treatment over the other, patient preference should guide selection of the treatment (American Psychiatric Association, 2006; American Psychological Association [APA] Presidential Task Force on Evidence-Based Practice, 2006). Because meta-analytic reviews indicate comparable outcomes for psychological and pharmacological therapies for most disorders, including anxiety and mood disorders, the unavoidable conclusion is that most patients are not engaged in their preferred treatments. The result, according to the research evidence (reviewed earlier), is higher premature termination, lower client satisfaction, and poorer treatment outcomes.

THE BROADER CONTEXT OF PERSONALIZATION

In ongoing treatment, it is not just preferences that can be accommodated. Rather, seasoned practitioners adapt to their patients in a multitude of ways. Even the most manual-bound psychotherapist in a fixed-duration randomized controlled trial (RCT) will evidence responsiveness by reacting differently to, say, a patient who is highly oppositional as compared with a compliant one (B. C. Chu & Kendall, 2009; Hatcher, 2015; Stiles et al., 1998). To this point, we have presented the evidence on preference matching as a separate, stand-alone activity, but every experienced therapist knows this is rarely the case in clinical work. These adaptation methods never act in isolation from the broader psychotherapy context, including relationship qualities such as empathy, collaboration, or support. Nor does it seem clinically possible to adapt psychotherapy in meaningful ways to the distinctive client and not routinely ascertain her feedback on the therapeutic process.

In our clinical teaching, we are frequently asked about the additive benefits of simultaneously matching psychotherapy to two or more patient characteristics. "What happens when you match therapy to preferences and other client features together?" Alas, we do not know for certain because empirical research has not kept pace with clinical reality. To our knowledge, only a couple of studies by Larry Beutler (2011) have investigated the effects of concurrent matching on two client qualities. Those results indicate added benefit, but no definitive answers are available yet (Norcross & Wampold, 2019).

Table 2.2 summarizes the meta-analytic research on personalizing psychotherapy to seven transdiagnostic patient characteristics (including preferences, as reviewed previously) compiled by an Interdivisional APA Task

TABLE 2.2. Summary of Meta-Analyses on the Efficacy of Treatment Adaptations and Relational Responsiveness to Patient Transdiagnostic Characteristics

Patient characteristic	No. of studies (*k*)	No. of patients (*N*)	Effect size (*d* or *g*)	Consensus on evidentiary strength
Attachment style	32	3,158	0.35[a]	Promising but insufficient research to judge
Coping style	18	1,947	0.60	Probably effective
Culture (race or ethnicity)	99	13,813	0.50	Demonstrably effective
Therapy preferences	51	16,269	0.28	Demonstrably effective
Reactance level	13	1,208	0.78	Probably effective
Religion and spirituality	97	7,181	0.13–0.43	Demonstrably effective
Stages of change	76	21,424	0.41[b]	Probably effective

Note. Adapted from *Psychotherapy Relationships That Work: Volume 2. Evidence-Based Therapist Responsiveness* (3rd ed.), by J. C. Norcross and B. E. Wampold (Eds.), 2019, Oxford University Press. Copyright 2019 by John C. Norcross and Bruce E. Wampold.
[a]Represents correlation between pretreatment security attachment and psychotherapy outcome; more secure attachment predict better treatment outcomes.
[b]Represents correlation between pretreatment stages of change and psychotherapy outcome; patients further along the stages experience better treatment outcomes.

Force (Norcross & Wampold, 2019). The evidentiary conclusions in the last column represent the consensus of an expert panel composed of 10 judges who independently reviewed and rated the research evidence. They evaluated the meta-analytic evidence for each adaptation/responsiveness method on the following criteria: number of empirical studies, consistency of empirical results, independence of supportive studies, magnitude of effect size of the adaptation method, evidence for a causal link between adaptation method and treatment outcome, and the ecological or external validity of research. The panel classified relationship elements as demonstrably effective, probably effective, promising but insufficient research to judge, or important but not yet investigated.

The meta-analyses employed the weighted d or g, standardized mean differences between two treatments or conditions—in this case, the difference between the conventional or nonadapted therapy and the adapted or matched therapy. In all of these analyses, the larger the value of d, the higher the effectiveness of the specific adaptation or tailoring. As a reminder, a d of .20 in the behavioral sciences is generally considered a small effect, .50 a medium effect, and .80 a large effect (Cohen, 1988).

Personalizing psychotherapy to a client's racial/ethnic culture, religious or spiritual identity, and, of course, therapy preferences will demonstrably improve treatment outcomes, and doing so to clients' coping styles, reactance levels, and stages of change will probably do so as well. Correlational research relating patient attachment security to psychotherapy outcome is promising, but there are not yet any prospective matching studies (Norcross & Wampold, 2018). Qualitative studies and a handful of uncontrolled quantitative studies suggest that attending to patients' gender identity and sexual orientation may also prove efficacious, but the absence of controlled studies did not permit meta-analyses (Norcross & Wampold, 2018).

The meta-analytic effect sizes in Table 2.2 range from 0.13 to 0.78 (a range of small to large effects) and average about 0.50 (a medium effect). Compare them with the 0.0 to 0.20 average effect sizes for the differential efficacy of one bona fide psychotherapy over another for a particular mental disorder (Wampold & Imel, 2015). That's why the Interdivisional APA Task Force confidently concluded, "Adapting psychological treatment (or responsiveness) to transdiagnostic client characteristics contributes to successful outcomes at least as much as, and probably more than, adapting treatment to the client's diagnosis" (Norcross & Wampold, 2019, p. 330).

Adapting treatment to patients' race/ethnicity and religion/spirituality was deemed demonstrably effective, with results that are particularly impressive. For race/ethnicity, the researchers analyzed 99 studies involving

13,813 patients (Soto et al., 2018). The mean effect size of .50 in favor of clients receiving culturally adapted treatments demonstrates that "cultural fit" works. Likewise, religious/spiritual-adapted psychotherapy resulted in a greater improvement in clients' psychological ($g = 0.33$) and spiritual ($g = 0.43$) functioning compared with nonadapted psychotherapies (Hook et al., 2019).

In another example, Edwards and associates (2019) conducted a meta-analysis of 13 RCTs investigating the effectiveness of matching therapist directiveness to the client's reactance level. Their meta-analysis found a weighted mean *d* of .78. This is a medium to large effect size, as shown in Table 2.2. In concrete terms, this effect size indicates that matching versus not increases success rates by 18% to 20%. These effect sizes translate into happier and healthier clients.

Research has determined that several matching methods work but has not yet pinpointed which particular adaptation method works best for any single patient (Norcross & Wampold, 2019). To some extent, it depends on the magnitude or strength of the effect size of the adaptation. To some extent, it depends on the salience that the client accords to that particular dimension or personal identity (e.g., race or ethnicity, gender, religion, sexual orientation). And to some extent, it depends on the clinical context and treatment goals. In all instances, success will largely depend on therapist flexibility and monitoring the client's experience of the intended responsiveness (Bohart & Wade, 2013; Levitt et al., 2016).

As the evidence base on personalization matures, we will know more about its effectiveness for particular circumstances and conditions. In "quant speak," we will know more about their moderators and mediators (Norcross & Wampold, 2019). In individualizing to preferences, for example, we have seen that personalizing to substance abusing clients proves not as effective as with other disorders (Swift et al., 2019). In adapting to culture (Soto et al., 2018), the researchers discerned in their moderator analyses that the single most effective adaptation was to use the client's native or preferred language. Moreover, the more cultural adaptations used in treatment, the larger the effect size.

Amid the torrent of meta-analyses and their limitations, let us not lose the overarching message: Multiple meta-analyses establish that personalizing treatment to preferences produces multiple benefits. Early research, in addition, suggests that adapting treatment simultaneously to several transdiagnostic client characteristics improves success even more. Take a mindful moment to consider the direct practice implications: Adapting therapy to the entire person improves success and decreases dropouts; the power of responsiveness exceeds that associated with Treatment Method A for Disorder Z. This constitutes not clinical lore, not gut intuition, but established fact (Norcross & Wampold, 2019).

META-ANALYTIC REVIEWS ON SHARED DECISION MAKING

Dozens of meta-analyses have also been conducted on the effectiveness of shared decision making (SDM), a practice that, as we saw in Chapter 1, is closely related to preference assessment and accommodation. These meta-analyses have largely been conducted on medical care—for example, SDM in pediatrics (Wyatt et al., 2015), surgery (Knops et al., 2013), and obstetrics (Dugas et al., 2012). Despite this difference, their findings are relatively consistent with those on preference accommodation in psychotherapy.

Overall, in terms of patient engagement and satisfaction, SDM interventions have been found to reduce treatment dropout, to increase patients' satisfaction and active involvement with their care, to improve patients' feelings of self-efficacy and self-management, to increase patients' knowledge about their condition and treatment options, and to enhance professionals' communication with their patients (The Health Foundation, 2012; Makoul & Clayman, 2006). Importantly, these findings seem to extend to disadvantaged groups (Durand et al., 2014), although a recent systematic review of SDM research in the United States found that the literature still lacks representation of minority populations (Perez Jolles et al., 2019). In terms of treatment outcomes, there is some evidence that SDM leads to improved health status, but there are also studies that show no such effect (The Health Foundation, 2012).

More recently, researchers have begun to examine the effects of SDM with mental health disorders. An initial 2010 review identified two rigorously conducted studies, both in Germany: one of inpatients with a diagnosis of schizophrenia and one of primary care patients with depression (E. Duncan et al., 2010). The depression study found that the SDM intervention increased patients' levels of satisfaction and involvement, and the schizophrenia study found that SDM patients had greater knowledge about their disorder at discharge. However, the SDM interventions were not found to improve clinical outcomes in either study.

A more recent meta-analysis (Stovell et al., 2016) sought to determine whether the implementation of SDM would lead to greater treatment-related empowerment for people with psychosis. Eleven controlled trials met the inclusion criteria and were subjected to meta-analysis. Primary outcomes were indices of patient empowerment and objective coercion (compulsory treatment); secondary outcomes were treatment decision-making ability and the quality of the therapeutic relationship. Small beneficial effects of SDM were found on increased empowerment (six RCTs; $g = 0.30$) and trends for SDM leading to reduced use of compulsory treatment over 15 to 18 months (three RCTs; relative risk [RR] = 0.59). No clear effect was found for SDM improving the quality of the therapeutic relationship (eight RCTs), but the data were heterogeneous. In short, for people suffering with psychosis, the implementation of SDM improves patient empowerment and may reduce involuntary treatment in the future.

Engagement and retention are particular challenges in substance use disorders. Friedrichs and colleagues (2016) sought to evaluate, via systematic review, the effectiveness of patient preferences and SDM in the treatment of substance-abusing clients. They located 25 trials encompassing 8,729 patients. The studies, in toto, found that patients with substance abuse disorders prefer to be actively engaged in treatment decisions, and matching patients to their preferences generally resulted in a reduction of substance use. But, as was also found in Swift et al.'s (2019) meta-analysis, the power of accommodating patient preferences was smaller in substance abuse populations than other mental health disorders.

In summary, although there have not been a large number of SDM studies published in mental health yet, the emerging evidence suggests that the positive effects of SDM are comparable to those documented in non-mental health patient groups (Patel et al., 2008). As well as improvements to patient satisfaction and engagement, as described previously, SDM increases treatment adherence and facilitates greater use of evidence-based practices (Trusty et al., 2019). Evidence of these positive effects is also supported by qualitative research, which we summarize in the next chapter. For policy, ethical, and practical reasons, therefore, partnering with clients in their treatment trajectories proves increasingly important.

IN CLOSING

In recent years, on both sides of the Atlantic, enthusiasm for personalized mental health care has blossomed. We see it among practitioners, researchers, and national funding priorities that increasingly emphasize precision psychotherapy and individually tailored treatments to optimize outcomes (Hong et al., 2019; National Health Service, 2016; National Institute of Mental Health, 2015). Like the legendary procrustean bed, one-size-fits-all treatments are widely seen as ineffective, inappropriate, and perhaps (as we argue in our next chapter) unethical.

Decades of controlled research and meta-analytic reviews now scientifically support what practitioners have long known: Different clients prefer and require different treatments and relationships. In the traditions of evidence-based practice and SDM, psychotherapists can create a new, responsive psychotherapy for each distinctive patient and their unique situation. Adapting care to patient preferences—along with other transdiagnostic characteristics—is effective in strengthening the therapeutic relationship, reducing premature termination, and improving psychotherapy success. This body of research provides a convincing starting point for the systematic assessment, and honoring, of patients' favored ways of working.

As one final example, in consulting with a large mental health organization, we were constricted in the telephone intake to adding a few brief questions about treatment preferences. We decided to inquire of every patient calling for behavioral health services, "Do you have a strong preference for a practitioner of a particular gender, sexual orientation, or language?" and "Do you strongly prefer medication, counseling/therapy, or both?" Consistent with the research, simply asking these questions increased patient satisfaction with the initial telephone screening (by almost a full point on a 5-point scale) and increased the probability of clients showing up for their first appointment. Respectfully and collaboratively inquiring about client preferences can exert dramatic effects on their treatment experiences. It is something for clinicians, of all orientations and professions, to prioritize.

3
THE CLINICAL EVIDENCE

Without clinical expertise, practice risks becoming tyrannised by evidence.
—David Sackett (founder of evidence-based medicine)

A foundational premise of evidence-based practice (EBP) holds that research alone will never suffice to make a clinical decision. Indeed, the straight extrapolation of controlled research to practice does not qualify as EBP. Such a linear approach lacks clinical sophistication, sensitivity, and real-world application. Clinicians understandably rail against such naivete and deride it as untenable "cookbook practice."

In practice, determining the optimal plan for a given patient constitutes a recursive process. Alongside asking "What does the research tell us?" we must always inquire "What is available and realistic? What does the clinician believe fits this context?" and a host of related questions. And so on, until we secure a seamless blend, a practical integration of best research, clinical expertise, and patient characteristics (Norcross et al., 2017).

https://doi.org/10.1037/0000221-003
Personalizing Psychotherapy: Assessing and Accommodating Patient Preferences,
by J. C. Norcross and M. Cooper

In the words of George Eliot (the pen name of Mary Ann Evans) in the novel *The Mill on the Floss*, "We have no master-key that will fit all cases." We must make treatment decisions, like Eliot's moral decisions, by "exerting patience, discrimination, and impartiality" and insight earned "from a life vivid and intense enough to have created a wide, fellow feeling with all that is human."

In this chapter, moving from the best available research, we consider the clinical evidence for personalizing psychotherapy. We examine, in order, the ethical imperative of incorporating patient preferences, the EBP requirement and process to do so, and the inextricably related value of cultural adaptations. We then consider some common pitfalls of the practitioner perspective and the probable mechanisms of action for the salubrious effect of honoring patient preferences. The chapter closes with an extended clinical case demonstrating the efficacy of preference accommodation.

THE ETHICAL IMPERATIVE

Even if assessing and accommodating clients' preferences had no discernable benefits on the outcomes of psychotherapy (and, as we have seen, it does), there would still be a powerful ethical argument for doing so. Indeed, with respect to shared decision making (SDM), some see the ethical case as more compelling than the research or "instrumental" one (The Health Foundation, 2012). This is for several reasons.

First, preference assessment and accommodation conveys a deep respect for our patients and their ways of seeing and understanding their worlds. The ethical codes of all mental health professionals contain the core principle of according dignity to the people with whom we work (American Psychological Association [APA], 2017; British Association for Counselling and Psychotherapy, 2018; Koocher & Keith-Spiegel, 2016). If we are not interested in our patients' preferences, or willing to engage with them, we are implicitly conveying that we do not value their understandings of what they want and need.

Second, assessing and accommodating our clients' preferences means respecting their rights to be autonomous, self-governing agents, another core principle of all professional frameworks (Koocher & Keith-Spiegel, 2016). Patients are provided with an opportunity to decide, in collaboration with their psychotherapists, how their treatment should proceed—it is not something done to them by an external force. As the slogan of the consumer movement goes, "Nothing about me without me."

Third, attending to client preferences is a means of "valuing each client as a *unique* person" (emphasis added; British Association for Counselling and Psychotherapy, 2018). It is a recognition that our clients are not uniform, machine-made products, but individualized beings with distinctive wants and needs. When we ask a patient, "What do *you* want from psychotherapy?" we implicitly communicate that their preferences may not be the same as another client's preferences. We recognize and respect their difference.

Such honoring of differences is not only crucial at the individual level but also at the cultural one—and across other sociocultural divides. A White male psychotherapist, for instance, who does not ask his female Pakistani client about her particular preferences for treatment, may end up imposing certain Eurocentric or androcentric (i.e., male-centered) assumptions. When we ask, we share power. We move away from a comparatively authoritarian, expert-led stance towards a more egalitarian and democratic one. This proves particularly important in working with clients who are already in positions of social disadvantage; that's probably why therapist positive regard or affirmation is even more effective for patients of color (Farber & Doolin, 2011). Rather than compounding feelings of powerlessness, we help such marginalized clients feel that their views can, and should, matter: that they have the right to determine their own pathways towards change.

To summarize, practitioners must honor patient preferences as part of their ethical duty. It is integral to respecting our clients' views, their autonomy, their individuality, and their intersecting cultural differences. Conversely, practitioners not identifying and accommodating their client strong preferences (unless clinically or ethically contraindicated) are acting unethically. Period.

THE EVIDENCE-BASED PRACTICE REQUIREMENT

Evidence-based practice (EBP) has a long past in medicine but a short history in mental health. The long past entails hundreds of years of effort to base medical practice on the results of solid research and experience. The short past of EBPs in behavioral and mental health traces back to the 1980s, originally in the United Kingdom, and then gathering steam in Canada, the United States, and now around the globe (Norcross et al., 2017). Many trace the early stirrings of the movement back to the United Kingdom and Archie Cochrane's (1979) article calling on medicine to assemble critical summaries of the scientific approaches that have proven effective according to randomized clinical trials. Cochrane and others contrasted EBP with *expert-* or *authority-based practice*, the latter lacking in solid research support and typically resulting in less effective health care.

The EBP movement initially concerned medicine—*evidence-based medicine* (EBM)—but quickly spread to other health professions, including behavioral health and addiction treatment. Thus, much of the vocabulary, for better and for worse, has come from the pioneering effort in EBM.

Adapting a definition from Sackett and colleagues (2000), the Institute of Medicine (2001) defined EBM as "the integration of best research evidence with clinical expertise and patient values" (p. 147). APA Presidential Task Force on Evidence-Based Practice (2006) and other mental health professions borrowed this foundation and expanded it, defining EBP as "the integration of the best available research with clinical expertise in the context of patient characteristics, culture, and preferences" (p. 273).

Several core features of EBPs become manifest in this definition (Norcross et al., 2017). First, EBPs rest on three pillars: available research; clinician expertise; and patient characteristics, culture, and preferences. By definition, the wholesale imposition of research without attending to the clinician or patient is not EBP; conversely, the indiscriminate disregard of available research is not EBP. Second, the definition requires integrating these three evidentiary sources. The integration flows seamlessly and uncontested when the three evidentiary sources agree; the integration becomes complicated and contested when the three sources disagree (see Chapters 6 and 8). Third, compared with EBM, the patient assumes a more active, prominent position in EBPs in behavioral health and addictions. "Patient values" in EBM rise to the status of "patient characteristics, culture, and preferences" in behavioral health EBPs.

The critical take-home here is that EBP, properly defined, requires the integration of patient preferences and culture into mental health treatment. It is not a luxurious add on or a clinical option; it proves necessary.

THE VALUE OF CULTURAL ADAPTATIONS

The global EBP movement and the incorporation of patient preferences are inextricably tied to cultural adaptations, in several ways. For one, patient cultures (along with characteristics) are embedded with preferences in the very definition of EBP. For another, a client's culture, inclusively defined, interacts invariably with their preferences. For still another, these factors constitute different ways of personalizing mental health care. Although researched independently, studies on preference accommodation and cultural adaptation aim for the identical result: tailored therapy to the unique person. For a final, both the accommodation of culture and preferences prove effective in improving outcome and lowering dropouts.

As introduced in Chapter 2, a recent meta-analysis showed the positive benefits of culturally adapted treatments (Soto et al., 2018). The most frequent methods of adaptation used clients' preferred language, incorporated cultural content/values, and matched clients with therapists of similar ethnicity or race. Cultural fit works; like preferences, it is not only an ethical and EBP mandate but also a scientific fact. Note, also, that common methods of cultural adaptation overlap with strong preferences as well. We suspect there is much "shared variance" in attending to culture and preferences. And the good news is that the more cultural accommodations are used, the larger the effect size (Soto et al., 2018). That is, more personalizing leads to greater patient improvement.

We frequently invoke the notion of *cultural humility* in assessing and accommodating patients' cultural preferences. It is, at root, an interpersonal stance that is other oriented rather than self-focused, characterized by respect and lack of superiority toward an individual's cultural background and experience (Hook et al., 2013). In multiple studies, client-rated perceptions of their therapist's cultural humility were positively associated with a strong working alliance and improvement in therapy. Notably, the therapist's self-rating of cultural competence bears no systematic relation to therapy success (Soto et al., 2018). Privileging the client's cultures, values, and preferences is what matters. That is the deep synergy, in philosophy and procedure, between cultural adaptations and preference accommodations.

THE PATIENT PERSPECTIVE

Assessing and accommodating clients' preferences is a means of respecting their autonomy and choices. A survey of over 12,000 patients in the National Health Service of England and Wales, for instance, found that 86% of respondents expressed a preference for at least one aspect of their therapy, such as the time of day of appointments, venue, or gender of therapist (Williams et al., 2016). When it came to type of treatment, over 50% had a particular preference. Interestingly, clients from marginalized social groups—females, nonheterosexuals, and non-Whites—were more likely to have preferences for particular aspects of their psychological treatment, supporting the point that preference accommodation and assimilation may be of particular value to these groups.

These findings have received support from SDM research. Most individuals do want to participate in decisions about their physical and mental care (Benbassat et al., 1998; Trusty et al., 2019). When patients are given a choice between a wholly active role (informed choice) and a wholly passive role (paternalism), the midpoint of shared and collaborative decision making is generally favored over either extreme. This is particularly the case for patients who are healthier, more educated, female, young, and not from minority ethnic groups (countering the earlier findings). In a qualitative study of clients' experiences of SDM in *pluralistic* psychotherapy (a collaborative integrative approach), most clients said that they felt comfortable engaging with this process and that it led to them feeling recognized as individuals (Gibson et al., 2020).

Of course, not all patients want to be involved in decisions about their psychological treatment or have strong preferences about how it proceeds. Around a third of the clients in the study of pluralistic therapy said that they felt "daunted" by being asked to take part in decision discussions (Gibson et al., 2020). In another qualitative study, one patient complained,

> As a client, I felt like she would ask me how the session had been for me at the end of every session as a kind of mini-review and I just felt totally, like, put on the spot, and still trying to process whatever we had been talking about. (Andrew, 2011)

As we emphasize throughout this book, tailoring needs to be tailored to the patients themselves: Some want more of it, some want less. Generally, however, most patients are either positive about the process of preference assessment and accommodation or relatively indifferent to it. Very few, as with the client quoted previously, show a strong dislike of it. Hence, there is substantial clinical support (in addition to the research evidence) for assessing and accommodating clients' preferences unless indicated otherwise.

PITFALLS OF THE PRACTITIONER PERSPECTIVE

Clinical expertise converges with empirical, ethical, cultural, and patient perspectives in guiding practitioners to customize therapy to their clients' strong likes and dislikes. There is a lengthy tradition in clinical work of SDM, ongoing collaboration, patient autonomy, and empowering clients. Fundamental skills of behavioral health practitioners include eliciting treatment priorities, establishing consensus on treatment goals, assessing cultural identities of importance, sharing the pros and cons of the alternatives, considering the socioeconomic resources, collaborating on the way forward, and continually monitoring progress toward the goals.

Mental health professionals, as a group, are dedicated to individualizing psychotherapy and are interested in learning how to do so more effectively. After all, who can argue against personalizing treatment to the individual in ways that demonstrably improve outcomes? It is like prizing Mom and apple pie. Not surprisingly, the therapeutic relationship and matching clients to therapists and therapy emerge as among the most desired skills that clinicians want from psychotherapy research (Tasca et al., 2015).

Practitioner-friendly translational research proves both prescriptive and proscriptive; it tells us what works and what may not. Of course, we could just reverse the effective adaptations identified in the meta-analyses (Chapter 2). Thus, for instance, what does not work is ignoring the client's cultural background or their stage of change. With respect to preferences, we can also identify some therapist actions that prove generally ineffective, perhaps even hurtful, in psychotherapy (Norcross & Wampold, 2019).

Imposing the Procrustean Bed

We should avoid the crimes of Procrustes, the mythological Greek giant who would cut the long limbs of clients or stretch short limbs to fit his one-size iron bed. We should not be imposing a Procrustean bed onto unwitting consumers of psychological services. Psychotherapists ought to be adapting to clients, not the converse (Norcross & Wampold, 2019).

Assuming We Already Accommodate Client Preferences

Given the dedication many of us have to individualizing psychotherapy, it may be easy to assume that we are already sufficiently engaged in preference work. Why do more? The research shows, however, that there is clearly room for improvement. Approximately a third of clients coming into National Health treatments in England and Wales, and who had a preference for a particular treatment, felt that they were not given adequate choice (Williams et al., 2016). Similarly, almost 90% of people with schizophrenia reported that they felt only partially involved or completely uninvolved in their choice of treatment (SANE, 2014). SDM research has consistently shown that "doctors, nurses and other clinicians often think they are sharing decisions more than their patients do" (Coulter & Collins, 2011, p. 33).

Presuming That Asking Is Not Needed

"Of course, I respond to any requests my clients make, so why do I need to ask?" For some clinicians, a tailored approach to psychotherapy may mean being open to any preferences that clients, themselves, express: "If clients want something, they'll ask." The problem here is that it does not consider the inevitable power dynamic that exists in the psychotherapeutic dyad, however "person-centered" the clinician may feel themselves to be. Research has demonstrated that clients are constantly "deferring" in treatment to their clinicians (Rennie, 1994). They may feel, for instance, that they do not have a right to ask, that the clinician knows best, or that their therapist will become annoyed with them and terminate treatment if they say what they would like. To break through these barriers, psychotherapists need to actively invite clients to state their preferences and make it clear that these are welcome contributions. Assuming this will happen rarely suffices.

"Intuiting" What Clients Want

A related danger is therapists assuming or intuiting that they know what clients want, without specifically asking. Alas, the research shows that there are many gaps here, and often our felt sense is not an accurate indicator of what clients want or need. Later in this chapter, we see an example of this phenomenon, when I (MC) had an "intuitive" sense that the client needed to talk about her current anxieties, but the client—quite rightly—recognized that she needed to explore more deeply her past. Developing the capacity to recognize and draw on our intuitive, embodied understandings is an essential clinical competence. But so too is the capacity to stand back from these feelings and recognize them as a single and limited source of information on how best to proceed with clients.

Cultural Arrogance

Psychotherapy is inescapably bound to the cultures in which it is practiced by clinicians and experienced by clients. Arrogant impositions of therapists' cultural beliefs in terms of gender, race/ethnicity, sexual orientation, and other intersecting dimensions of identity are culturally insensitive and patently less effective (Norcross & Wampold, 2019). By contrast, therapists' expressing cultural humility and tracking clients' satisfaction with cultural responsiveness markedly improves client engagement, retention, and eventual treatment outcome (Soto et al., 2018).

Flexibility Without Fidelity

Therapist flexibility to the patient's preferences, values, and cultures helps to ensure that psychotherapy "fits" the patient but not necessarily that the resultant treatment has any research support. Having emphasized here the benefits of treatment adaptation, we caution against ignoring the research evidence on the effectiveness of psychological treatments. Focusing solely on accommodating without addressing the client's problems or distress will not prove optimally effective (Yulish et al., 2017). While the research supports adaptation in many cases, the research also recommends fidelity to treatments as found effective in controlled research. We need to balance flexibility with fidelity (J. Chu & Leino, 2017).

Singular Adaptations

In the quest to personalize psychotherapy, some psychotherapists become enamored with one form of matching and apply that to virtually every patient who crosses their path. They become convinced that a single adaptation— be it the patient's preferences, diagnosis, culture, or stage of change—is the exclusive means of tailoring treatment to a successful outcome. However, the research convincingly demonstrates that many adaptations work. We must guard against imposing the Procrustean bed when we adapt psychotherapy; one size, even in adaptation or responsiveness, never works for all clients (Norcross & Wampold, 2019).

DO CLIENTS WANT WHAT THERAPISTS WANT?

Another potential pitfall when working with client preferences is assuming that our clients want what we want. It is tempting to conclude, for example, that because we despise psychotherapists giving us advice or reassurance, that our clients will despise that too. Perhaps you have watched painfully as a fellow professional deposits her treasured life learnings onto an unwitting and unprepared client. This is particularly problematic when what has worked for that professional proves radically different from what works for the patient. Psychologically, this is known as the *false consensus effect*, in which we see our own behavioral choices and judgments as more common than they actually are (Mullen et al., 1985; Ross et al., 1977).

There is plentiful research on the treatment preferences of mental health professionals. Psychotherapists often opt for psychodynamic or psychoanalytic therapies for their own treatment (Norcross, 2005). Integrative and humanistic therapies have also proven popular. Historically, behavioral therapies have been less favored, even among behavioral therapists (Geller et al., 2005; Lazarus, 1971). As clinicians, we tend to prefer more insight-based, reflective approaches. By contrast, research with laypeople has suggested that they tend to have more of a preference for cognitive behavior therapy (Bragesjö et al., 2004).

To investigate this question in more depth, we (Cooper, Norcross, et al., 2019) quantitatively compared two samples of laypersons (N = 228, 1,305) with one sample of mental health professionals (N = 615); the first layperson group was an online convenience sample, and the second layperson group was a large and demographically representative sample of U.K. and U.S. citizens. Comparisons were made on the four dimensions of the Cooper–Norcross Inventory of Preferences (C-NIP): Therapist Directiveness versus Client Directiveness, Emotional Intensity versus Emotional Reserve, Past Orientation versus Present Orientation, and Warm Support versus Focused Challenge (see Chapter 5, this volume, for details on the C-NIP).

Robust differences were found between laypersons' and professionals' preferences on two of the four dimensions (Cooper, Norcross, et al., 2019). Specifically, laypersons favored more therapist directiveness and less emotional intensity in psychotherapy than did the mental health professionals. The magnitude of the differences was large, with Hedges's gs of 0.92 and 1.43 on the directiveness scale for the therapists compared with the convenience and representative laypeople, respectively, and 0.49 and 1.33 on the emotional intensity scale for the same comparisons, respectively.

Figure 3.1 presents boxplots for these two scales for all three samples; mental health professionals and laypersons clearly differ in their preferences. Laypersons typically enter therapy preferring that their therapists focus on specific goals, provide structure, teach skills, and take the lead far more than the therapists themselves prefer. At the same time, compared with professionals, laypersons typically favor less emotionally intense sessions—that is, less frequently being encouraged to express strong feelings and with less focus on the therapeutic relationship. On our two other dimensions (preferences for past orientation and for warm support), however, there were no significant differences.

These findings confirm earlier evidence that clinicians and clients systematically vary in what they, themselves, prefer in psychotherapy. This does not mean that clinicians will necessarily impose their own preferences onto clients, but it does point to the risk. The take-home message is that we need to reflect carefully on our own psychotherapy preferences and what we would want and expect from psychotherapy (and the C-NIP measure

FIGURE 3.1. Differences in Preferences for Therapist Directiveness and Emotional Intensity Between Mental Health Professionals and Representative (Lay Sample 1) and Representative (Lay Sample 2) Samples of Laypeople

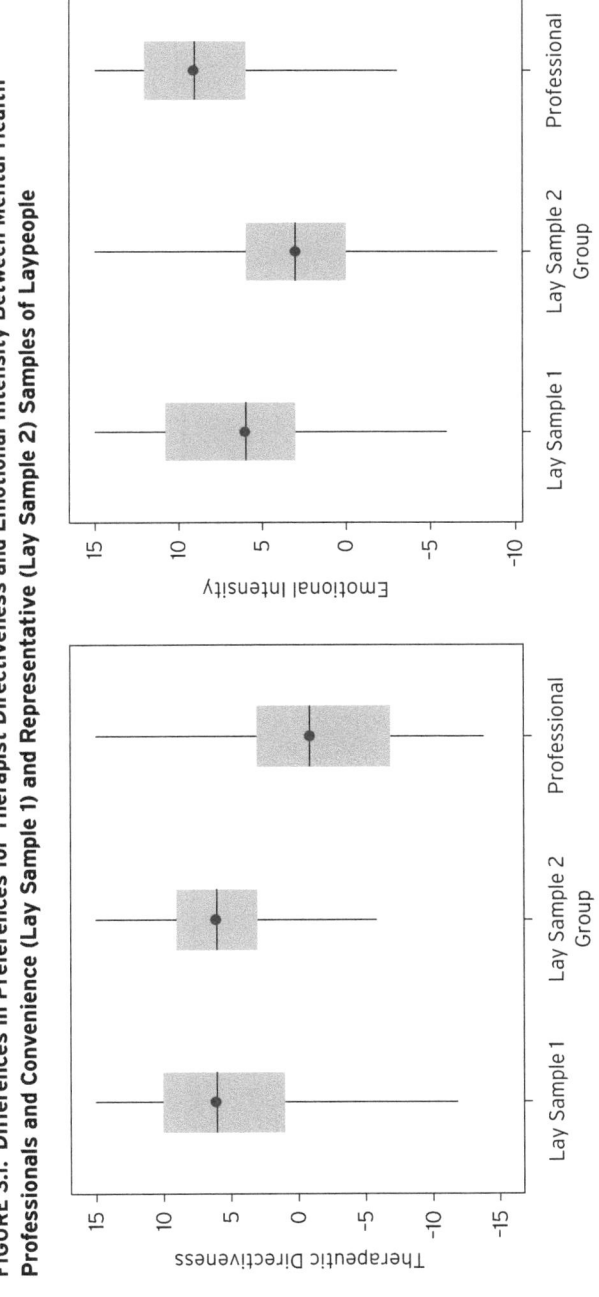

Note. Reprinted from "Psychotherapy Preferences of Laypersons and Mental Health Professionals: Whose Therapy Is It?," by M. Cooper, J. C. Norcross, B. Raymond-Barker, and T. P. Hogan, 2019, *Psychotherapy, 56*(2), p. 211. Copyright 2019 by American Psychological Association.

is one structured means of doing that). We will then be more skilled in noticing when we might project our treatment desires onto our patients. That awareness will optimally lead us to separate our preferences from our clients' preferences, to stand back and listen to what our clients themselves are actually asking for.

PROBABLE MECHANISMS OF ACTION

While it is empirically clear that assessing and accommodating clients' strong preferences enhances treatment outcomes and client satisfaction (Chapter 2), it is unclear precisely why that is the case. Three main mechanisms of action have been proposed (McLeod, 2012): matching effects, choice effects, and alliance effects.

Matching Effects

When we think about why preference assessment and accommodation prove effective, *matching effects* are probably the immediate thing that comes to mind. This starts from the premise that clients, at least to some extent, "have a fairly good sense of what they like and what works and does not work for them" (McLeod, 2012, p. 26). Hence, a treatment guided by these insights is likely to provide the patient with more of what is helpful to them and less of what is unhelpful. If a client knows that they find behavioral experiments useful or that they cannot profit from mindfulness exercises, matching therapy to those desires is likely to maximize benefit.

An illustration of this matching comes from Jong-Su, a young Korean man, who attended 13 of 24 allocated psychotherapy sessions before dropping out. Jong-Su's clinician had been trained in a relatively nondirective, person-centered approach. At the endpoint interview, Jong-Su said,

> The thing that I found quite difficult was just the lack of structure. I'm not very open so it takes a lot for me to . . . talk. Which is why I need someone to question me or—I don't know what I should be talking about. I know problems I have but I don't necessarily know how to get round those or how, you know—solutions for that.

The clinician had been asked to assess and accommodate Jong-Su's therapy preferences, but his capacity to do so seems to have been limited. Jong-Su said,

> We did talk about it, and then there would be a little bit of structure, and then it would be back to talking about random things again and no structure. . . . After, I think, the second review [at Session 10], where I realized that nothing was really going to change. It wasn't [his] style—it didn't really feel important.

In this situation, it would probably have been more effective for the clinician to be open with Jong-Su, early on in the treatment, about the difficulties that he would encounter matching to Jong-Su's preferences and to discuss together alternative options or referral.

The catch here, of course, is that matching effects will only prove helpful to the extent that clients know (and can communicate to the clinician) what works and does not work for them. For instance, although Jong-Su thinks he needs structure and direction, it may be that what will help him is the kind of unstructured, nondirective treatment that his person-centered therapist could provide.

Research does indeed support the claim that what patients say they prefer is not necessarily or automatically an expression of what will prove best for them. Instead, patients, at different times, will vary in their levels of *motive congruence* (the degree of agreement between "implicit" and "explicit" motives; Thrash et al., 2012). A more nuanced understanding is needed of when clients may have most (and least) insight into what they want.

Probably the most accurate mediator of motive congruence is how familiar an individual is with a particular domain (Lichtenstein & Slovic, 2006). Say you frequented a restaurant that served Chinese or Italian food. If you eat these foods fairly regularly, then you would have a good sense of what you like. But if you visited a restaurant that served Kazakhstani food, it might be much more difficult to choose between *kazy*, *kuyrdak*, or *baursaks* (assuming you do not know that cuisine well). Under these conditions, the congruence between what you opt for and what you prefer is a lot more tenuous—ending up, for instance, with a plate of sheep's chopped heart, liver, and kidneys boiled in oil (that's the *kuyrdak*!). Transposed to the psychotherapy domain, the key point is that a client experienced in psychotherapy will, in all probability, have more knowledge of what does (and does not) work for them than a novice client.

Other factors also determine how well patients know their own treatment wants. Motive congruence is, on average, higher in self-determining individuals whose early environment supported the development of self-determination by meeting their basic needs for autonomy and relatedness (Thrash et al., 2012). Motive congruence is also higher in individuals who are more sensitive to their bodily states and less monitoring of others' expectations.

In summary, one of the principal ways in which preference assessment and accommodation can benefit clients is by increasing the likelihood that they will receive treatments that genuinely match what proves most helpful to them. However, as Arnold Lazarus (1993), founder of technical eclecticism and a great advocate of personalization, wrote, "It would be naïve to assume that patients always know what they want and what is best for them, and that clinicians are those advised to slavishly follow their clients' scripts" (p. 409). Rather, as psychotherapists, we need to find ways of navigating between the Scylla of paternalism (where we ignore clients' preferences) and the Charybdis of informed choice (where we hand over responsibility to them). The answer, to a great extent, lies in *dialogue*: inviting clients to express their preferences, exploring with them the rationale and robustness of these choices, sharing our own views, and reviewing and revisiting, where appropriate, the decisions that have been made.

One final point, going back to Jong-Su: Perhaps his problems were rooted in an external locus of control, and a nondirective therapy would have benefited him most in the long term. But the problem was that his therapy was framed and delivered in such a way that he did not stick around long enough to discover that. This is why the powerful effect of preference accommodation on reducing dropout is so compelling (Swift et al., 2019): We cannot help our clients if they are no longer in treatment with us. Even when we do not agree with our client's treatment preferences, it usually makes sense to align with them so that a therapeutic alliance develops. As the work progresses, we can then introduce more of our own perspective and explore together optimal ways of working.

Choice Effects

Although matching effects may appear the most obvious reason why preference accommodation works, the research evidence is probably stronger for *choice effects*. This refers to the impact of clients feeling that they have some say in, and control over, how their treatment is rendered.

An ingenious study demonstrated this effect (Handelzalts & Keinan, 2010). Students suffering from test anxiety were treated with either progressive muscle relaxation or cognitive behavioral modification, but under three different conditions. In the first, they were allocated to their preferred treatment and made aware that this was the case. In the second, they were also allocated to their preferred treatment, but they were told that the allocation was random. The third condition was a waitlist control. Students in the first group, those who thought that they had control over their treatment, did better than those in the second group, even though the latter were just as likely to receive their preferred intervention. These results show that the perception of choice can have a positive impact, irrespective of whether there is an actual match between preferences and treatments.

Why might this be the case? First, the perception of having a choice and exercising it can bring about positive affective responses. Research shows that the act of choosing is associated with increases in positive affect and the activation of dopaminergic reward mechanisms in the brain (Caplandies et al., 2018; Leotti & Delgado, 2011; Sharot et al., 2009). A sense of control is considered one of the most fundamental human needs by many psychological theorists (e.g., Geers et al., 2013; Powers, 1973), and the accommodation and assessment of clients' preferences in psychotherapy may contribute towards it. Consistent with this, one study found that around half of clients described the experience of SDM as "empowering" (Gibson et al., 2020). One client said it "gives you a bit of power over the things that have caused you pain and, obviously if you're in therapy because of them you feel powerless."

Second, feeling involved in making a choice can lead to increased positivity, engagement, and motivation toward that chosen option, which can then lead to improved treatment results. Participants given a choice between two analgesics experienced less anxiety about a painful task (putting their hand in cold water) than those not given a choice (Rose et al., 2012). Empirical support that choices can affect attitudes goes back to research into cognitive dissonance theory (Festinger, 1957), which argued that people justify their choices by realigning their beliefs, evaluations, and commitments to suit.

Again, though, research points to factors that moderate and mediate the impact of choice effects. First, as with matching effects, there is domain familiarity: Clients who know more about psychotherapy may feel more respected and valued by being given a choice than those unfamiliar with this domain (Caplandies et al., 2018). Second, the number of choices available impacts the effects of those choices: While a few may feel empowering, too many may lead to feelings of overwhelm, confusion, and ego depletion (Geers et al., 2013). Third, the importance of the choice to the person can moderate its effects (Fox et al., 2016): A patient taking psychotherapy seriously may appreciate choices more than one who feels "made to go." Fourth, a person's desire for control impacts choice effects (Burger & Cooper, 1979): how important it is for the individual to be independent and autonomous (Fox et al., 2016).

In short, research has shown that the experience of having, and making, a choice can be salutogenic (i.e., well-being enhancing), and this may account for some of the positive benefits of preference assessment and accommodation. The evidence also indicates that these effects are likely to be highly dependent on situational and patient characteristics. If a client is familiar with psychotherapy, is presented with a manageable number of (relevant) choices, and likes to be in control, then it seems likely that preference accommodation will evoke positive feelings and a greater commitment to the treatment. But with unfamiliar, overwhelming treatment choices—for a client who does not want to be in control—the effects may be different.

Matching effects and choice effects may act in relatively independent ways. So, for instance, a patient might feel empowered by being offered a choice of psychotherapies but end up choosing an approach that, in fact, is not particularly helpful to them.

Alliance Effects

Offering clients choices may also help them feel a stronger bond with their clinicians and more aligned on the goals and tasks of their psychotherapy. These increases in the *therapeutic alliance*, as has been consistently demonstrated in the research, may then lead to improved treatment outcomes (Flückiger et al., 2018; Zilcha-Mano, 2017). In contrast to matching and choice effects, this is a more indirect route (or mediational effect) through which preference accommodation leads to positive benefits (Winter & Barber, 2013).

Danielle, introduced in Chapter 1, illustrates how the assessment and accommodation of client preferences strengthen the alliance. What might it mean for Danielle that she could tell her psychologist that she needed more physical distance between them and that this preference was heard and accommodated? Her smile when I (JCN) put a coffee table between us suggests that she experienced my accommodation not only as a clinically preferable configuration but also as an expression of my understanding and respect. Approximately half the clients in the qualitative study of SDM in psychotherapy specifically reported feeling "listened to and understood" as a result of this process (Gibson et al., 2020).

Preference assessment and accommodation also have the clear potential to enhance agreement on the tasks and goals of therapy, the two other critical elements of the therapeutic alliance (Bordin, 1979). This concerns clients' perception that they and their psychotherapists are "on the same page." Through preference discussions, the client often concludes that their therapist knows what they are trying to achieve in treatment and how they will most like to get there.

Having said that, the relation between preference work and the alliance is almost certainly bidirectional. Have you ever been to a restaurant and had the menu "thrown" at you by a surly waiter who then stands over your seat as you anxiously try to decide what to eat? However compelling the choices may be, if they are not offered in the context of a warm, welcoming, and caring alliance, their benefits are likely to prove limited. As Borrell-Carrió and colleagues (2004) wrote, "It is entirely possible to advocate for shared decision making without challenging the notion of the cold technician" (p. 579). Preference assessment and accommodation, then, can be understood as one factor with the potential to contribute to the quality and strength of the alliance—but only one.

These three mechanisms of action—matching effects, choice effects, and alliance effects—probably account for the documented effectiveness of preference assessment and accommodation. In fact, it would be instructive to conduct additional studies (although, perhaps, of questionable ethics) that disentangle the effects of feeling that one's preferences were being taken on board (choice) from the actual matching to those desires (match) with and without a strong personal relationship with the practitioner (alliance). Whatever their relative contribution to the preference effect, all three will prove instrumental in performing preference assessments and accommodations, and all three will guide our recommendations in forthcoming chapters.

GABRIELLA: A CLINICAL EXAMPLE

We conclude this chapter with a clinical case to illustrate concretely how the assessment and accommodation of client preference add value to psychotherapy—for both the client and the clinician.

"When I first heard about psychoanalysis," said Gabriella, her eyes starting to smile, "I thought. . . ." Gabriella, introduced at the start of Chapter 1, stopped midsentence and broke into a hearty laugh. It was the first time in her initial meeting with me (MC) that her expression of anxiety and concern had broken. "But then," she continued, "I read Jung . . . and I found good things, so I really—it's something effective."

Gabriella was describing her treatment preferences using the C-NIP, described in Chapter 5. Gabriella had already indicated a strong activity preference for exploring her childhood: "It's just my idea," she said, that "the problems come from the past, but if you, the therapist, see there's a problem in a different aspect, of course, then I am open to that."

Gabriella indicated two other strong preferences. First, she wanted me to facilitate emotional intensity:

> I am a 27-year-old adult—and I'm like a 60-year-old when I'm thinking things through. But when I'm getting into my problems and feelings, I'm 5 or 6 years old! It's this age gap. Anger, and all those childish feelings when people push me. So that's why, emotion-wise, I need to face my deep, deep down troubles.

Second, Gabriella wanted to be challenged "because I am very good at playing games some times. I make assumptions, so the therapy has to be quite pushy to stop me just making up what I think is going on."

"I wonder if that will make you angry at times," I said, referring back to Gabriella's earlier description of feeling pushed.

"Yes," agreed Gabriella, "but this is the kind of a safe environment for me to have that anger displayed."

Gabriella had some familiarity with the psychotherapy domain after six sessions of behavioral counseling in her late teens. She said that she understood the point of the exposure work—"being told to go into the situation that stresses you for 90 minutes"—and had found it somewhat helpful. At the same time, she came away feeling angry towards her therapist:

> I didn't see any care in his work. And I felt that if I was in that position, somebody came to me and told me their problems, I would feel a bit "show some emotions," "show some care." I didn't feel that way. He wasn't unkind, he wasn't. . . . I want more of a mother figure, someone nurturing.

What brought Gabriella to psychotherapy? In her assessment session, based at a public mental health clinic that offered up to 24 sessions, she described her fear when away from her house: "I worry I might do something weird in public." She particularly hated walking down the street and felt that she was being watched and silently criticized. "I shouldn't think about what others say," she said, "It's more important what I think about myself." She added that it was hard to build relationships because she was feeling defensive all the time, just waiting for another attack. Gabriella also wanted to develop her capacity to make a positive contribution to the world. Since being in the United Kingdom, she had worked as a receptionist at a small local hotel and wanted to secure more meaningful work. She had been studying, part time, for a degree in politics, and her ambition was to work as a researcher in the Houses of Parliament. Gabriella's scores on psychometric tests confirmed that she was experiencing moderately severe anxiety and mild levels of clinical depression.

Sessions 1 to 3: Gabriella's Childhood

As Gabriella requested, in the first three sessions of psychotherapy, I invited her to talk through her childhood. She had been raised in the center of a Spanish city, the daughter of a taxi driver and a textile maker. Her maternal grandmother was the matriarch of the family artisanal clan, famed for their vibrant fabrics. Their small business, however, had been gambled away by the maternal grandfather, and Gabriella's mother had been reduced to piecework for local tourist companies. Because her mother worked, Gabriella spent most of her youth being brought up by her maternal grandmother, "Abuela." She was a fiercely loving woman, protective of Gabriella, and, in Gabriella's eyes, Abuela favored her above all her cousins. In the battles between Abuela and Gabriella's father, who resented the grandmother's dominance in the family and her antipathy towards men, Gabriella consistently took her beloved Abuela's side.

Gabriella described herself as a nervous and sensitive child, following Abuela around the family shack, never letting her out of sight. School proved a shock to her, and the downfall of the family was the subject of much teasing by her classmates, many of whom came from more bourgeois origins. Gabriella struggled to speak in class, afraid that her voice would give away her family's class background. "I knew the answers," she said, "The words bubbled up in me. But I was like in the middle of a war zone in my head. Fighting to push them up and push them down."

Then, one day, the words came out, but not at all like Gabriella imagined: "When I spoke, it was a strange, garbled sound that came out of my mouth—nothing at all like the words in my head." Flushed with shame, Gabriella tried harder and harder to correct herself, to retract her words, but dug herself deeper and deeper into a hole of self-abasement. "Probably," she said, "it lasted only a few moments. Maybe no one noticed too much. No one said anything. But it wrenched me out from inside."

Homelife, too, was difficult for Gabriella at this time. Her Abuela developed angina and eventually died from a heart attack. Gabriella became teary as she described this in Session 2 but said that she did not feel ready to talk more about it. Her parents' relationship at this time deteriorated rapidly. Her mother was becoming increasingly, almost obsessively, desperate to earn money for the family, while her father was becoming more disengaged from the home. The parents fought frequently. Eventually, Gabriella felt that she could not bear it any longer and came to Britain to escape the "madness" around her. Initially, she enjoyed living in London and had a varied social life with Spanish compatriots, including several lovers. But over time, she kept more to herself, working long shifts to send money back to her parents and avoiding romantic dates because of the stress of going out: "It just feels too much these days. I can't put my shoes on without starting to shake."

Session 4: Review

Session 4, a preplanned review session, was scheduled before the Easter break. Gabriella asked whether, for that session, she and I could do something "lighter." We discussed what that might be and agreed that we would look at methods for helping Gabriella calm herself. I taught Gabriella breathing exercises and took her through a progressive muscle relaxation procedure, ending with the visualization of a safe space. Gabriella found it helpful, and I said that I would bring in a workbook that could help Gabriella learn other visualization methods.

My formulation was that, at this point, it might make sense to focus on Gabriella's current anxieties. However, Gabriella indicated that she wanted to delve more into her past. In particular, she wanted to talk more about her Abuela. To me, a solid relationship seemed to be developing with Gabriella. Gabriella's scores on the Working Alliance Inventory (Horvath, 1992), towards the top of the scale, suggested that she, too, was experiencing a good working relationship.

Sessions 5 to 7: Family Business

At the start of Session 5, I invited Gabriella to talk more about her Abuela. Nervously, Gabriella began. She described her grandmother's history: the trauma and loss she had experienced as a result of her husband's gambling, the persecution brought about by being on the losing (Republican) side in the Spanish Civil War. Despite all that, she had been there, ferociously, for Gabriella.

And what had the child Gabriella done? She described stories of playing outside as she could hear her Abuela moaning in pain, following her schoolmates to the park for cigarettes when her Abuela had asked for help with shopping. Was she any better, she asked, than the grandfather who squandered their livelihood and then abandoned his wife? Gabriella cried as she described how much her grandmother must have suffered and how she wasn't there for her. "And I'm afraid," sobbed Gabriella, "that she'll never forgive me for abandoning her—wherever she is now." Mindful of her desire for emotional intensity, I invited Gabriella to "breathe into the pain." "I'm afraid that she is suffering still," Gabriella said. "I want to know that she forgives me, that she still loves me. I should have been there for her."

I suggested a two-chair exercise, imagining her Abuela, sitting opposite, talking to her. "What would she say to you?" I asked, "What would she really think?" Gabriella took a few moments to reflect. "She'd want to know that I was OK," she said, exhaling with relief. "OK," I said, gently repeating the words of her grandmother, "I'd like to know you are OK?"

"And she would want to know that I wasn't suffering," added Gabriella.

"Would she forgive you?" I asked.

"Yes, she would forgive me—like that," said Gabriella, snapping her fingers. "She knew human beings. She's seen so many things, so many ups and downs." Gabriella smiled, "She would be telling me off for feeling bad. She'd be saying, 'Get on with life.'"

At the start of the next session, Gabriella said that she had been quite upset and shaken during the week, with many images and memories of her Abuela. But she said that she wanted to continue focusing on their relationship. I, knowing her preference for emotional intensity and past focus, readily agreed. Gabriella visualized being with her grandmother and this time imagined her Abuela holding her and telling Gabriella that she loved her. She imagined, too, telling her grandmother that she was sorry: "You were my true mother," she said to her, weeping. Gabriella was intensely emotional throughout and, at the end of the session, described the work as "very helpful": "I am feeling huge relief addressing this issue so openly."

In the following session, Gabriella asked to focus on her father and her anger towards him for never being there. "He still just takes and takes," she complained. She and I explored ways in which Gabriella could be more assertive with him and other people in her life. "Like the other two sessions," Gabriella wrote on her session feedback form, "This has been a huge wake-up call for me for my real feelings."

Sessions 8 and 9: The Here and Now

Session 8 began with reflecting together on the next steps for the therapy:

MC: I was wondering what it might be useful to focus on. We talked about—last week we talked about your father, and we started talking about anger, and at some point, we need to talk about your anxieties and focus on that. [*Gabriella:* Yes, yes.] Have you thought about where would be good to go for this session?

GABRIELLA: Um . . . I feel a bit easier about the past, and I want to jump somewhere in the future. But is that a misleading feeling? I don't know. Am I running away from a difficult past? I'm not sure. Until now, what we've done in the past has had a huge, huge impact. It's the first time I feel like I can talk about Abuela without almost crying. Like a choking feeling. And what is your opinion about it? What do you think is best, what is your sense?

MC: I think at some point, we need to talk about your anxieties. [*Gabriella:* Yeah.] Um, maybe we can start today by talking about that. [*Gabriella:* Yes.] And that doesn't mean we can't go back to talking about the past.

GABRIELLA: Yeah, yeah, I think it's good. I'm ready [*laughs*].

MC: I know you are. Well, where's a good place to start? At the moment, how are those particular anxieties?

Gabriella replied that her anxieties had improved slightly since starting therapy but went on to describe the fears that were crippling her ability to lead "a normal life." She expressed how, for instance, at college lectures, she would have the same internal battles between talking and keeping silent: a terror of exposing herself. Gabriella described how her fears had made it impossible for her to engage in beloved activities, such as going out dancing. "I feel the eyes on me," she said, "I know people are judging me, criticizing me. I *know* they aren't, but I know they are."

"I wonder," I asked, "whether you also have some of the same fears here with us?" Gabriella had indicated on her C-NIP that she was keen to explore the here-and-now therapeutic relationship, and I thought that it could be helpful to bring Gabriella's anxieties into the immediate relationship. Sheepishly, Gabriella nodded in agreement.

She talked about her anxiety that I might "kick her out of therapy" if she challenged me or blurted out something ridiculous and be mortified. "So how do you think I see you?" I asked. Gabriella described her fantasy or projections: that I was bored by her, just on the borders of accepting her—which was why she had to be the "perfect client."

I listened, reflected, then asked Gabriella whether she would like to know how I did experience her. Gabriella nodded. I shared that, in reality, I valued our time together and looked forward to seeing her each week. After a pause and a smile, I asked Gabriella how it was to hear that.

To my surprise, Gabriella then described aspects of my clinical behavior she found quite annoying and disappointing. Where was the workbook that I had promised her? Why was I so disorganized, and why did I seem to be stifling yawns during the sessions? Gabriella related that she worried I was not giving my best or preparing as much as I could: This was her "golden shot," and she wanted to make the most of it.

I listened respectfully and answered that I would take on board her feedback. I also raised with her the idea of idealizing versus demonizing and that perhaps she harbored either high expectations of people or a lot of disappointment, with little grey area in between. I introduced to Gabriella the Kleinian concepts of "schizoid" and "depressive" positions and the aim of moving from the former, black-and-white divisions to the latter, more integrated—albeit more disappointment-filled—ones. Maybe it was important, I said, that Gabriella could experience disappointment with me. After the session, Gabriella wrote, "Talking about our relationship was a huge help. I still feel uncomfortable about it, however at least I have the courage to say how I feel about our relationship as therapist and client."

That week, I secured the workbook for Gabriella and sent it to her.

Gabriella began Session 9 saying that she was worried she had upset me, to which I replied that she had not. Was that true? Probably not entirely. I recognized that I was experiencing some hurt, but given Gabriella's desired goals (tackling her anxieties and dealing with her past), I did not believe it would prove relevant or helpful to disclose these countertransferential feelings.

Gabriella then expressed her deep fear of letting people down, especially those who had been caring and kind to her. It was a real challenge, she said, to allow herself to trust that someone would be there for her. Towards the end of the session, I introduced the transactional analysis (TA) concept of the adapted child—that Gabriella had a part of her that was desperate to please and comply with others. "What would it be like," I asked Gabriella, "to feel like you are good enough now—just as you are? Not perfect, not awful, but good enough."

Sessions 10 to 24: Getting Out

Session 10 was a second scheduled review session, and Gabriella and I decided that we should return to focusing on Gabriella's current anxieties. Drawing on cognitive methods, we made a list of Gabriella's negative automatic thoughts, such as "Other people think I'm crazy," and examined more adaptive and realistic alternatives (for instance, "No one really cares that much what I do"). We subsequently looked at what Gabriella might do to get out of the house more, and I introduced the idea of paradoxical intentions: deliberately trying to do the thing you are most scared of. "What would happen," I asked, "if in a social situation, you would say things that were bizarre or weird—if you tried to make yourself do it?" Gabriella laughed, but the thought that she could shout out, in public, "Sod David Cameron!" (the British prime minister) or "Up the Gunners!" (her favorite soccer team, Arsenal) took the sting out of her fears. Then she tried it in session. She switched her inner voice from, "Oh my god, I might say something terrible" to "What the hell; let's think of the worst thing to say."

Gabriella indicated that she was finding this focus on her current anxieties helpful. As a consequence, in Session 13, Gabriella and I agreed to construct an exposure hierarchy. It ranged from "Standing in their front garden on a quiet day" (least scary) to "Sitting in a full, but deadly quiet, church" (most scary). Over the following weeks, Gabriella worked through them one by one.

In the final weeks of therapy, Gabriella and I explored her fears of flying, her religious beliefs, and her sadness at ending therapy. Gabriella also spoke more about her excitement for her politics degree and how it could draw on her natural skills of astuteness—even paranoia, she joked. By the end of treatment, Gabriella evidenced a reliable reduction in her anxiety level and enhanced well-being. Repeat administration of the psychometric instruments confirmed that both her anxiety and depression were now in the nonclinical range.

General Discussion

The case of Gabriella demonstrates how the ongoing process of preference assessment and accommodation guided a successful course of psychotherapy. Assessment of Gabriella's wants at the start of treatment meant that the treatment was immediately oriented to a productive area of work: her childhood. At Session 4, when I thought it was time to "move on," a scheduled reassessment of her preferences instead led us to remain focused on—and dug deeper into—her childhood losses, guilt, and anger. This was, perhaps, the most useful element of her psychotherapy: assisting Gabriella in letting go of some guilt towards her grandmother and reconnecting to Abuela's love and care. My knowledge that Gabriella strongly preferred emotional intensity and challenge enabled me to keep Gabriella to task here, even though Gabriella herself sometimes showed resistance or avoidance. Inviting Gabriella to express her preferences regularly also helped and empowered her to raise genuine concerns about the therapy and the therapist, such as not receiving the workbook she had been promised.

As a pluralistic, integrative therapist, I drew on concepts and methods from a range of theoretical orientations—person centered, cognitive, behavioral, interpersonal, and TA—but what tied them together was a constant centering on their SDM. At the start of treatment, as well as the start of each session, when things were not clear, I used the opportunity to ask Gabriella to see what she wanted to do. This was not about abdicating responsibility to Gabriella, but about inviting her into a collaborative discussion to genuinely consider together what was best for her. Here, Gabriella was a wise, thoughtful, and constructive contributor, and so was I. Two experts—one in psychology, one in Gabriella's life—giving their best to assist Gabriella in determining and obtaining positive ways forward.

IN CLOSING

In a technology-fueled world (Greenberg, 2016), there is a pervasive tendency to standardize, industrialize, and mechanize what we do with our clients. Psychotherapists would do well to heed the ancient wisdom in the Hippocratic Oath (modern version): "I will remember that there is art to medicine as well as science, and that warmth, sympathy, and understanding may outweigh the surgeon's knife or the chemist's drug." It goes on, "I will remember that I do not treat a fever chart, a cancerous growth, but a sick human being." Reaffirming the human element and attending to the patient's totality in psychotherapy stem from this moral commitment, as well as robust evidence.

We have seen, in this chapter, the ethical, evidence-based, and cultural arguments for personalizing. Exploring the mechanisms by which preference assessment and accommodation can bring about affirmative outcomes also directs our clinical activities. At the same time, in looking at these three mechanisms, and focusing on a clinical example, we start to appreciate the nuances and complexities of working with client preferences. Asking clients what they want from treatment, and accommodating it, can be choice empowering, alliance strengthening, and match promoting, but, in select circumstances, it may also be experienced as overwhelming.

Onwards, then, to the next chapters on assessing and integrating clients' preferences into treatment, always with the understanding that this skilled and sensitive process requires the best from us as clinicians.

4 ASSESSMENT OF CLIENT PREFERENCES

O World, Thou choosest not the better part!
It is not wisdom to be only wise,
And on the inward vision close the eyes,
But it is wisdom to believe the heart.

—George Santayana

So, how do you actually go about assessing clients' preferences? In this chapter, we provide a hands-on guide to assessing client preferences in a reliable, relational, and effective way—tailored to the individual patient. This will then form the basis for Chapter 5, which focuses specifically on preference assessment using measures, and Chapter 6, which considers the integration of client preferences into psychotherapy.

https://doi.org/10.1037/0000221-004
Personalizing Psychotherapy: Assessing and Accommodating Patient Preferences,
by J. C. Norcross and M. Cooper

YOUR OWN SCOPE OF PRACTICE

Before proceeding, we need to consider an essential prior question: What is your own *scope of practice*? By this, we mean what are you (a) competent to offer clients and (b) willing to offer them? Assessing and accommodating clients' preferences, as we repeatedly emphasize in this book, is not about being a jack-of-all-trades, nor is it about becoming a chameleon who changes colors to whatever a patient requests. Rather, it is about offering flexibility within defined parameters—and, when necessary, being willing to refer patients elsewhere (see Chapter 6).

An in-depth discussion of what it means to be competent in a particular treatment, or therapy activity, is beyond our purview. However, for our purposes, you may find it useful to identify the treatment models/theoretical orientations that you believe you are competent to deliver, as well as the range of therapist activities. Regarding the latter, below is a list of the 20 most commonly used methods across diverse psychotherapies (Thoma & Cecero, 2009). Which of these are you competent to provide?

1. Trying to understand the world from the client's point of view (empathy).
2. Providing unconditional positive regard.
3. Challenging maladaptive or distorted beliefs.
4. Being congruent and genuine.
5. Reflecting patient feelings.
6. Planning and encouraging alternative behaviors.
7. Assisting the patient to work through or apply insights to a range of life situations.
8. Training the client to notice how thoughts, assumptions, or beliefs cause different emotional responses.
9. Calling attention to here-and-now awareness.
10. Teaching clients to recognize and change their shoulds, oughts, and musts.
11. Scheduling or encouraging pleasurable activities.
12. Offering positive reframing to help a person change their narrative about a person or situation.
13. Facilitating the discovery of a sense of meaning and purpose.
14. Exploring early childhood experiences.
15. Encouraging the client to examine their own role in the maladaptive family system.
16. Encouraging the client to be present to, or authentic with, the therapist.

17. Exploring and interpreting emotional problems in terms of problematic interpersonal relationships.
18. Giving the client feedback about their present-tense body language or manner of speech.
19. Facilitating client focusing on present-tense internal feelings and sensations.
20. Empathizing with what the client is avoiding or minimizing.

Assessing your willingness to offer diverse treatments and activities is also an important consideration and, to some extent, independent of your competence to do so. For example, you may be a certified cognitive behavior therapy (CBT) practitioner but no longer desire to offer that therapy. For those treatments and activities you are competent to deliver, as identified above, now ponder whether there are any that you are not willing to provide. Alternatively, there are probably treatments and activities that you are not yet competent to provide but would like to develop skills to do so.

You may also find it useful to use the Cooper–Norcross Inventory of Preferences (C-NIP; see Chapter 5 and the Appendix; it can also be downloaded from www.c-nip.net/) to deepen an awareness of your scope of therapeutic styles. For each of the 18 dimensions presented there, circle the range within which you are (a) competent and (b) willing to provide. For instance, on Item 1, if you are skilled and content to focus on clients' specific goals but would not like to work in an entirely non-goal-focused way, then you might circle 3 through to −1. This exercise can prove valuable if you ask your clients to complete the C-NIP because it may identify areas of compatibility and incompatibility.

Another benefit of completing the C-NIP in this manner is that it underscores the psychotherapist's flexibility. Classical Rogerians, for example, will probably discover that they prefer working in a less directive manner, but they are both competent and willing to work in other ways in select situations, in the spirit of the person-centered approach. In fact, we have been playfully accused of using this exercise to demonstrate that the vast majority of mental health professionals are integrative in practice; very few of us are theoretical purists.

HOW TO APPROACH CLIENT PREFERENCES

Having sharpened your awareness of your own scope of practice, let us consider some general principles of assessing clients' preferences.

It's the Relationship, Stupid

As we saw in Chapter 3, preference assessment and accommodation need to be practiced in the context of a broader relationship. This frame is ideally a respectful, genuine curiosity to understand the patient's sense of what is likely to prove beneficial and what will not. It is an exciting, joyful process of codiscovery. For many of us, it is among our favorite parts of therapy: identifying and actualizing individual differences. The assessment is an invitation to dialogue—to dance, if you will—about what specifically might work for the other. It constitutes, in our view, an advanced form of empathic relating.

Without at least a modicum of that ambiance, the assessment itself will probably deteriorate into a sterile process of collecting more, irrelevant information. If it does, we implore psychotherapists not to bother with preference work at all. If clients' preferences are considered immaterial by the clinician, it is better to skip the "charade" of assessing them altogether.

We have taken of late to saying that "culture eats strategy," as the management consultant Peter Drucker put it. The relational and responsive character of psychotherapy frequently proves more powerful than a particular method, even one intended to be responsive. Thus, a key ingredient of preference assessment is the authentic desire to know the other, dialogue about their desires, and attune treatment responsively in that direction when possible. This is not merely an ephemeral, internal state of the therapist; it properly manifests in your behavior toward the patient—in twinkling eyes, a soft smile, a forward lean, a genuine invitation, or a verbal–nonverbal congruent desire to codiscover. Set your heart right; bring Santayana's "wisdom of the heart" to the encounter.

Some examples of *non*empathic introductions to assessing patient preferences are presented here. Lest you think we are confabulating these, they are taken, nearly verbatim, from recorded therapy sessions:

♦ [*Clinician audibly half-sighing.*] "Oh, and another thing. I am supposed to collect your preferences for psychotherapy. The Center makes us administer this questionnaire."

♦ [*After meeting the client for a total of 35 minutes.*] "I have a pretty good idea of what you want from counseling, so we can skip the usual questions on your preferences and get to it." [*Moves on without pausing for a client response.*]

♦ [*Sounding annoyed.*] "I don't know about you, but I hate doing these intake assessments. So just complete these forms quickly; the answers really don't matter for what we do anyway."

◆ "This is a measure created by one of my supervisors. He thinks it helps treatment." [*Client completes the C-NIP, clinician takes back the piece of paper, places it in the file, and then immediately finishes the mental status examination.*]

Invite Clients to Share Their Preferences

In this relational dance, we believe psychotherapists should "reach out" to their patients rather than assuming their patients will step forward with their wants. Inevitably, a power dynamic exists between patient and practitioner, and research shows the tendencies of clients to defer to their clinician (Rennie, 1994). Consequently, clients may feel uncomfortable or inhibited from sharing treatment preferences. For instance, they may think, "Surely it is not my place to voice my opinion here"; "If I ask for something that the therapist doesn't like, she may make me leave therapy"; or "I don't want to embarrass my therapist by making them think they're doing something wrong." Of course, these reactions may be furthest from our minds and lips, but clients—particularly those used to critical or defensive responses from others—may predict such responses and much worse.

Hence, it is rarely enough to respond empathically and acceptingly if clients do voice preferences. Rather, clients should be actively invited to say what they have strong likes and dislikes for—to be introduced to the idea that the psychotherapeutic process is one that they can shape and offer feedback on. Here are a few "openers" by which clients can be invited to voice their preferences:

◆ "Based on your previous experiences of therapy, what do you think will be useful here?"

◆ "What would you like in our work together? Do you have any sense of what might be helpful or unhelpful to you?"

◆ "I have been conducting and researching psychotherapy for 40 years, and we have learned the importance of tailoring or personalizing psychotherapy specifically to you. May I ask a few questions to identify your strong likes and dislikes for psychotherapy?"

◆ "Try this brief exercise. Close your eyes, breathe deeply a few times, and imagine in your mind's eye what you would strongly like to happen in here. What would I ideally do? What would I not do?"

◆ "Let's think together about how to reach your therapy goal. Which treatment method? What type of therapy relationship? What type of out-of-office activities—self-help, exercise, apps, and so on?"

Solicit Likes and Dislikes

Actively inviting clients to share their preferences may be particularly vital in identifying what they would strongly *dislike* in treatment—and, even more so, what they are strongly disliking now. For a client to say to a psychotherapist, for instance, "I don't find it helpful when you ask me to do homework" or "I wish you would say more in our sessions" may feel excruciatingly awkward. Many clients will need to be reassured, perhaps several times, that such "critical" feedback is welcomed—indeed, that the clinician welcomes it as part of their own learning and development. The "facts are always friendly," so to speak.

At the start of a review session, a few weeks into treatment, a counselor might say,

> So, we said, at the start of counseling, that we would review how things were getting on around this point. I wanted to ask you how you were finding therapy. Is it feeling helpful or not so much? And it would be good to know what's not working, as well as what is. Please do feel free to say about anything you don't like or that you'd want to be different. I know that can be difficult to say, and you might be worried a bit about hurting my feelings, but I promise that's fine with me. In fact, it's good for me to hear those things so that I can work on personalizing therapy to you.

Normalize Client Reactions to Preference Assessment

Although clients expect to be asked about their treatment goals, they are typically surprised when the clinician inquires into their psychotherapy preferences. Hundreds of our psychotherapy patients (and supervisees) have spontaneously exclaimed, "I was not expecting that!" or "Did not see that coming" or "I was not prepared for that question." A therapist can transform this novelty into a learning or therapeutic moment.

When patients respond with surprise or incredulity to the invitation, we take a number of tacks depending upon their reaction and clinical context. But we squarely put the emphasis on (a) normalizing their reaction then (b) leveraging it to distinguish psychotherapy from most health care. Normalizing responses do just that; for instance, "It is rare to be asked what you want"; "Your surprise is understandable and frequent; that's not how it's usually done"; and "Not expecting that one, huh? Doctors don't often ask what the patient wants."

We segue immediately into a brief explanation and, we hope, a corrective experience into how psychotherapy differs from most health care. That can be communicated in words and deeds. I (JCN), for instance, say something along the lines of

> Much of medical care remains rooted in the passive patient receiving treatment from an authority. But in here, in psychotherapy, we expect and cultivate an active patient working together to create the best treatment. I am an expert on behavior change and psychological growth, but you are the expert on you and your preferences. We will collaborate and work as a team to personalize or individualize therapy to you.

(Recall that the terms *personalize* and *individualize* were those most favored and intelligible to laypersons in our focus groups.)

If the client is a health care professional or familiar with the terminology, then I might add "Similar to precision or personalized medicine" and finish with "How does that sound to you?" or "How would that work for you?"

Be Part of the Dialogue

An active client does not require a passive clinician. Instead, he or she requires an active psychotherapist who can work in a dynamic, animated, and dialogical manner to reach the best treatment collaboratively. That's the meaning of *shared decision making* (SDM): facilitating the decision discussion, ensuring clients have space to voice their opinions, acknowledging their wants, and explicitly encouraging them to say what they want. The clinician asks questions and offers reflections that help the client, more clearly, articulate their preferences. It is an iterative cycle. For instance,

THERAPIST: So . . . you've said you want to work through how you're feeling about the end of your marriage. In your experience, are there ways that are more or less helpful in doing that?

PATIENT: It's good to have . . . space to talk. Definitely. [*Pauses*]

THERAPIST: So, by "space" you mean . . .?

PATIENT: Kind of . . . time. Not rushing, not feeling like I have to get it all out at once.

THERAPIST: So time, not a rush. No pressure.

PATIENT: Mm. . . . Just that someone—that they're not waiting for me to finish so that they can talk. That they want to hear.

THERAPIST: So in working together, what might help is me giving you the time not to feel any pressure about saying stuff. Not trying to rush in. Letting you take things at your own pace. Is that it?

PATIENT: Yes. . . . It's kind of something about letting me *feel* things. Really feel.

Here, we see that, as the clinician actively enters into dialogue with the client on strong preferences, further details and nuances emerge. The psychotherapist works with the client to bring these preferences out—just as they would with other aspects of their clients' perceptions or experiences.

Nearly all clients, in our clinical experience and our research studies (e.g., Gibson et al., 2020), welcome specific suggestions from the clinician on how to improve psychotherapy. This is not to say that clients are dismissive of their own understandings and perceptions: They believe they have much knowledge and insight into their preferences too. But they see the clinician as an expert in knowing *how* to apply those preferences, to transform general desires into specific practices.

This is consistent with SDM in medical encounters, which emphasizes the role of the clinician in sharing information with the patient about the available treatments, their likelihood of success, and potential risks (Hanson et al., 1997). Only the patient can know how different factors weigh for them—for instance, whether 6 months longer to live outweighs the pain of chemotherapy. But what the patient may not know, and what the health care professional can advise them on, is how painful that chemotherapy is likely to be or how much longer they may be likely to live with it. Equally, most clients do not come into psychotherapy knowing that two-chair work can be used to address intrapsychic splits or that motivational interviewing can be effective for substance abuse. Here, psychotherapists have a capacity and an ethical responsibility to share such valuable information.

Suggest Alternatives Through Scaffolding

A lasting lesson from our clinical experience and research is that it is rarely helpful to give clients a "blank sheet of paper" and inquire, "What do you want?" As the psychological research confirms, an extensive or unlimited range of options can prove overwhelming (Chapter 3). Rather, it is often better to describe a small number of options that clients can choose between—to *scaffold* possibilities—informed by the clinician's expertise on what might be most helpful to the client at that particular time. We saw this in the clinical example of Gabriella (Chapter 3), where I (MC) suggested specific techniques to work through guilt and grief with her grandmother (two-chair work) and then her current anxieties (paradoxical intention, an exposure hierarchy).

The following dialogue is with Debs, a middle-aged White woman experiencing anxieties and dysphoria. At assessment, Debs flagged a number of painful childhood experiences that she wanted to work through, but by Session 10, she felt ready to address her current anxieties head-on.

THERAPIST: It sounds like you're saying that you've got a sense of those things from your past being more resolved. Now you want to look specifically at tackling your anxieties.

DEBS: Yes, like being able to talk and do presentations at work without feeling like I'm going to crumple into a heap. If I'm going to progress, I know I'm going to have to do that.

THERAPIST: And do you have a sense of what we can do helpfully?

DEBS: I guess, perhaps, I could do more of saying things to myself—being more positive: "C'mon, stop being stupid. Put yourself forward."

THERAPIST: Yes, we could look at ways that you talk to yourself and perhaps see if there's helpful ways for you of doing that. There's also an approach that is quite helpful for people where we make a list of the things that you're scared of doing, from the least scary to the scariest, and then we could look at you trying to do them one by one. For instance, the least might be sharing your ideas with a small group of friends, and the most might be offering to do a talk to the whole board of directors [*both laugh*]. Any thoughts on what might be helpful there?

DEBS: I know that doing that list terrifies me, but I also know that I've got to sometimes just do things. I can talk myself around in circles and end up where I started. So—

THERAPIST: So, shall we give that a go, and we can see what it's like?

In suggesting options, clinicians might bear in mind two important points (Tompkins et al., 2013). First, as emphasized from the start of this chapter, only offer options that you are willing to meet. There may be a temptation to describe a range of abstract and ideal possibilities, rather than specific treatments or activities that you can competently offer the patient. Second, describe the options thoroughly and carefully so that clients have a meaningful understanding of what they are. To this, we can add a third point:

Present the alternatives with *decisional equipoise* (E. Duncan et al., 2010). That is to say, describe each in a genuinely balanced way, rather than suggesting that one of the options is "better" or more desirable than the other.

Compare the following "options" depicted by a therapist:

THERAPIST 1: Well, I guess we could try and explore your emotions using two-chair work, but, to be honest, most clients prefer just talking about them.

THERAPIST 2: Some clients find it helpful to explore their emotions using two-chair work, and others like to talk directly about them. Do you have a sense of what might work best for you?

Even if you do not think you are explicitly communicating your preferences to clients, you might still be doing so implicitly. Indeed, this is a repeated finding in the SDM research: What clinicians describe as "shared decision making" can be experienced by patients as a biased prompt in a particular direction (The Health Foundation, 2012). Offering decisional equipoise, then, requires clinicians to be consciously aware of their biases and to deliberately bracket them so that clients are genuinely free to make the choice that is right for them.

The exception is when the clinician does have a strong opinion based on clinical expertise or the research evidence that one alternative is more effective than another. Under such circumstances, it is nearly always best for the clinician to share this position with the client so that the different elements of evidence-based practice can be weighed against each other. We explore this process more fully in Chapter 6.

Be Confident

At its best, preference assessment communicates to clients that we are interested in their perspectives and value their unique desires. At its worst, however, preference assessment can communicate to clients that we have no clear idea of what might help them and that we are laying the responsibility for treatment success on their shoulders alone. Thus, questions about client preferences must be delivered confidently and positively, rather than in a pleading, befuddled, or apprehensive way.

I (JCN) learned the need to assess treatment preferences from a place of strength the hard way: in a humorous but unfortunate clinical interaction. A talented psychiatric resident was learning in supervision to identify her patients' treatment desires. We (JCN and the resident) discussed how to do so, and she felt confident enough in her abilities that we did not role-play or practice it in the supervision hour. Next time we met, she showed the videotape of her first attempt to gauge preferences with a middle-aged man seeking combination therapy (psychotherapy plus medication) for chronic depression. The videotape captured their interaction:

RESIDENT: My supervisor, Dr. Norcross, believes that your preferences for psychotherapy are important and can help improve our effectiveness. So, how do you think I can do psychotherapy best?

PATIENT: [*Cocks his head like a quizzical dog.*] Shouldn't *you* know how this works? Maybe I should be seeing Dr. Norcross instead?

The resident was mortified, and we were guilty of not ensuring that she was adequately prepared. Fortunately, 2 weeks earlier, we had practiced alliance rupture–repair skills, and she effectively handled the transgression with her patient thereafter.

Lessons learned in the baptism of practice! First, assess from a place of strength or confidence, not inexperience or "the supervisor said. . . ." Second, begin with the invitation or an orientation, which will include presenting the rationale for assessing preferences. Third, practice how to assess before venturing boldly into the consulting room.

Construe Assessment as an Ongoing Process

Treatment and therapist preferences may be one-off decisions made by the client that then determine the course of the psychotherapy. By contrast, as we saw in the case of Gabriella, within-treatment activity preferences may be elicited multiple times over the course of psychotherapy, as clients discover and evolve their preferences. Clients' preferences may change as a consequence of events in their lives, or they may become more knowledgeable about—and confident to express—their preferences. Do not take the client's first expression of preferences as a fixed and immutable truth. Rather, see it as the opening statements in a dialogue that will unfurl over the course of psychotherapy.

Tailor the Amount of Tailoring

Consistent with our emphasis on honoring client preferences, we do not require anyone to complete a preference assessment or measure. Should patients indicate that they are not willing, interested, or ready to do so, then we respect that decision. The assessment can be completed later or not at all.

At the risk of proceeding down a hall of mirrors, preference assessment and accommodation is likely to suit clients to different extents at different points in time. While, as a general rule, all clients should be asked about their strong preferences, they should not be pressured into expressing preferences if they are not willing or able to do so (Trusty et al., 2019).

In Chapter 3, we reviewed research showing that clients who have not had psychotherapy previously, who are more extrinsically oriented, and/or who have lower desires for control are the least likely to hold strong preferences towards their psychotherapy. However, probably the best way of gauging whether a client wants to be involved in decisions about their care is simply by asking them in an equipoisal way. For instance, "Some people really want to be involved in deciding how therapy should proceed, others really don't, and some people don't mind either way. There are no right or wrong answers here. How about you?"

Of course, when clients say that they do not want to be centrally involved in treatment decisions, the challenge is to find a balance between (a) accepting this and not pressuring them and (b) being respectfully persistent in communicating that we are genuinely interested in their views. A few follow-up questions usually suffice. But if those clients remain adamant that they have no strong preferences for therapy, it is likely better to move on, with the possibility of coming back to this at a later date. Novice clients, in particular, may require some experience of psychotherapy before they can render an informed opinion on their preferences.

It may also be helpful to "seek feedback from patients about their perceptions of involvement in decision making" (Trusty et al., 2019, p. 1213). A therapist might ask something along the lines of, "You have probably noticed that I often ask you at the beginning of sessions about what you'd like to work on, and I wonder how that is for you?" or "How are you finding our end-of-session reviews?"

WHAT TO ASSESS

Patients' strong likes and dislikes can be assessed across treatment, therapist, and activity preferences (Chapter 1). Think of it as a 2 × 3 grid (Figure 4.1): Strong likes and Strong dislikes down the vertical axis and Treatment preferences (e.g., cognitive behavior therapy vs. person-centered, psychotherapy vs. medication), Therapist preferences (e.g., male vs. female, straight vs. gay), and Activity preferences (e.g., high vs. low directiveness, homework vs. not) across the horizontal.

FIGURE 4.1. Matrix of Patient Psychotherapy Preferences

Strong likes			
Strong dislikes			
	Treatment preferences	Therapist preferences	Activity preferences

Based on this map, initial preference assessment might involve asking two open-ended questions: What do you strongly dislike or despise in treatment? What do you strongly like or desire? If psychotherapy has already been chosen as the primary or exclusive form of treatment, then those prompts can be modified to "psychotherapy" in place of "treatment."

There is no compelling research or experience to dictate whether one asks for likes or dislikes first. Some colleagues begin with the positive and seek the primacy effect of likes. Others begin with the negative and aim for the recency effect of likes. It is a matter of therapist preference and comfort.

These questions can be phrased in a variety of ways. A clinician, for instance, could ask what patients "despise" as that word conjures strong emotional meaning, as opposed to the more cognitive appraisal associated with "strong dislike." Some psychodynamic colleagues have taken to asking patients what they "despise and fear," which introduces an extra element.

Three recent patients articulated their strong likes and dislikes for psychotherapy:

♦ A therapy-experienced young adult: "I like activity and energy. My last therapist sat there and repeated back what I said to him. Please bring something to the table—ideas, methods, topics. And, no offense, but not much about your own life, OK?"

♦ A mental health professional in training: "Hmmm. Well, I know you are integrative because I wanted to avoid a 'true believer' type of therapist. So definitely not straight relational or cognitive or humanistic. I prefer that you give me space to talk and feel. Lots of support, too; I am probably a bit needy. Given the local area, I am concerned about confidentiality—not about you, really—but seeing other therapists or students coming into your office."

♦ A client new to counseling: "Not sure. Haven't given it that much thought. . . . But I know that I don't want medication, and my cousin said I should ask for some DBT stuff. I looked it up online but not sure it is for me." Later in the session: "You know, that was nice that you asked what I wanted. It gave me a warm, fuzzy feeling that you see me as, well, me."

Expect to hear the full range of human desire and loathing.

For some treatment episodes, asking these two questions will prove sufficient. In many cases, mental health professionals do not have the time or luxury to assess on a wider range of treatment preferences. Here, it is essential to attune therapy to two or three strong client preferences. This can make the most impact and maximize cost-effectiveness. In other cases, however, clinicians will want—or have the opportunity—to explore client preferences in a more comprehensive and detailed manner across the course of psychotherapy.

Either way, a useful precursor to exploring preferences is to ask clients about any previous experiences of mental health services and what they liked/found helpful or did not like/found unhelpful in this work. As reviewed in Chapter 3, domain familiarity is one of the best predictors of the effectiveness of preference accommodation. Hence, asking clients about these experiences yields valuable prognostic indicators of the probable value of honoring their preferences in this episode of care. Clients who have not had mental health treatment can still be asked about support from friends or family: What was helpful and unhelpful to them when eliciting support in these relationships?

Treatment Preferences

Having explored strong likes and dislikes at a general level, we typically explore the three preference categories. Questions about treatment preferences are most likely to be asked at initial assessment—or even on first contact—and their appropriateness will largely depend on the client's familiarity with the psychotherapy domain. Clients with an extensive history of therapy—perhaps they are even mental health professionals themselves—frequently have strong views on which treatment approach they want. By contrast, clients who are new to psychotherapy are often entirely unfamiliar with terms such as *psychodynamic*, *CBT*, and *existential*, such that asking questions in these areas may be baffling (at best) and shaming (at worst).

Accordingly, questions about treatment preference should be framed cautiously, and not assuming clients will know the range of options. Here are two examples:

♦ To a client who had not experienced therapy before: "There are different approaches to psychotherapy available, and I wondered whether you had an idea of which one might be more or less helpful to you? It's totally fine if you don't because lots of people wouldn't have a sense of that."

♦ To a client who has had therapy before: "I was wondering about your previous therapy. Do you know what sort of therapy it was? Did that work well for you? What was helpful and unhelpful about it?"

As the last question suggests, even when clients had psychotherapy in the past, they may not know the name of the specific treatment. But they probably know which specific in-session activities did and did not work for them (activity preferences). When clients do identify a specific treatment by "brand name," it is still worth following up with more questions about what they specifically liked or did not like, partly to develop a more nuanced understanding of their preferences, partly because the client may have misassociated treatment names with particular practices. More than once, we have encountered clients saying that they like "psycho-dynamic therapy" because it helps them focus on their present thoughts, or "behavioral treatment" because then they do not have to perform exposure exercises!

When clinicians offer specific, "brand name" therapies, they may wish to describe them here, during this natural point in the session. Some clinicians characterize this as presenting their treatment model or describing their therapy rationale. This can be done either verbally or using vignettes of different therapies. Here are two examples of written descriptions of treatments (adapted from E. Freire et al., 2015):

♦ *Person-centered counseling.* Counseling provides you with an opportunity to talk about what is troubling you so that you can explore your thoughts and feelings about it in a way that is not always possible with family and friends. Being listened to by someone who is not judging you, and who is trying to understand things from your perspective, can help you see things in a new light. The therapist will encourage you to discuss your experiences and express your feelings, but you will decide which topics you want to talk about and how much you want to say. This therapy aims to help you to feel more positive and confident about yourself.

♦ *Guided self-help CBT.* CBT teaches practical life skills that address many of the common problems faced during times of low mood or stress. It aims to help you identify any unhelpful patterns of thinking and responding that are worsening how you feel. With guided self-help CBT, you will have access to either an online course or short, practical books that teach these skills. You will also receive regular telephone support calls from an experienced support worker. The aim is to help you apply what you are learning and make helpful changes in your life that aim to boost how you feel.

Therapist Preferences

As with treatment preferences, therapist preferences are assessed prior to treatment commencing and often even before a first meeting. Unlike treatment and activity preferences, however, there is limited ability for the clinician to be flexible here: They cannot overnight change gender, ethnicity, or sexual orientation in response to clients' wants!

As a result, the assessment of therapist preferences is most relevant in settings where the client can select among several professionals. It is not uncommon, in a consumer-driven private-practice marketplace, for potential patients to try out or interview several therapists. These questions may also prove useful in routine practice for multiple situations: (a) intake or triage appointments when the assignment of therapists has not yet been determined, (b) initial intake with a particular therapist to determine whether that person is the optimal fit for that client, and (c) when arranging for a referral to another clinic or practitioner.

There is a wide variety of therapist characteristics that clients might be asked their preferences on. These include the clinician's

♦ gender,
♦ race or ethnicity,
♦ age,
♦ professional status (licensed/qualified or trainee),
♦ sexual orientation,
♦ religion or spiritual commitment,
♦ marital status,
♦ language(s), and
♦ life experience (e.g., whether they have experienced the same problems as the client—for instance, alcoholism or trauma).

When inquiring into preferences about the therapist, we recommend bearing in mind the possibilities of deference and impression management. A female Black client being assessed by a White male psychotherapist, for instance, may find it difficult to say that she would rather work with a Black woman. We are fond of saying to clients, "My professional commitment is to match you with the best therapist for you, even if that is not me." Patients may need reassurance and empowerment that they can express potentially "offensive" preferences. So in the example just mentioned,

> Do you have strong preferences for the kind of psychotherapist? I mean, would you prefer someone male, female, or other; a particular ethnicity or age; or other characteristics? I know it might be difficult to say to me, as an older White man, that you'd rather work with a younger therapist or a person of color, but I'm fine with it. I won't be offended, and it's much better that you express what you want and don't want now, at the beginning.

Like assessment of all types of preferences, it may prove effective to offer clients time to reflect on therapist preferences before responding. We have proposed that clients mull it over during that session or by email after the session, sometimes even at the beginning of the next session (when feasible). That ofttimes enables patients to express desires that may be uncomfortable for them to say to the therapist's face—and for some therapists to hear.

Activity Preferences

Activity preferences are likely to be assessed at both the start of treatment and throughout psychotherapy to the very end. These preferences include *client activity preferences*—what the client wants to do in treatment—as well as *therapist activity preferences*—what the client wants the clinician to offer. Given the vital contribution of client agency and engagement to treatment outcomes (Orlinsky et al., 2004), it is probably a good prognostic indicator if clients express activity preferences in terms of what they want to do, as well as what they want from their therapist. However, for clinical purposes, therapists benefit from some "translation" of client activity preferences into what this means clients want from them. Here is an example:

THERAPIST: You're saying that you would like to get to a place where you can be closer to people. Do you have a sense of how we can work together to help you get there?

PATIENT: In my last therapy, I talked a lot about my childhood and my relationship with my parents, and that gave me quite a lot of insights, but it didn't really change much of how my relationships go. So, I think that I'd like to focus on something more practical.

THERAPIST: So, perhaps helping you to focus on your current relationships and practically looking at what you might do differently. And what can I do helpfully in that?

PATIENT: I think exploring with me what I'm doing wrong. Like pushing me a bit to face some uncomfortable truths.

THERAPIST: OK. Encouraging you to go into ways that you relate that might be difficult to accept, maybe hard to face up to.

PATIENT: Yes. My last therapist was very positive about me, and I liked that, but it was too comfortable in some ways. I need someone to also point out the problems. I mean not in a judgy way, just honest.

THERAPIST: For me to be honest with you about the things I see you doing, that, perhaps, might not be helpful.

The range of activity preferences that can be collaboratively decided is virtually limitless (Papayianni & Cooper, 2018). To start with, we have the format and frequency of psychotherapy. Asking clients about any strong preferences in these areas, when flexibility is possible, contributes to a more collaborative and equitable therapy relationship. Areas for discussion can include

♦ modality of therapy: individual, couple, family, group, or some combination thereof
♦ platform of therapy: in person, videoconferencing, telephone
♦ number of sessions: short term or long term, open ended
♦ frequency of sessions: every week, every 2 weeks, every month, ad hoc
♦ length of sessions: 30, 45, 60, 90 minutes

Many other boundary and frame issues might be deliberated. For example, I (JCN) had the following conversation in my second meeting with a bright, funny, but also depressed teenager with attention-deficit/hyperactivity disorder (ADHD). I remember it plainly because of the young man's quick wit and because he was one of my all-time favorites (yes, of course, shrinks have their faves):

PATIENT: What should I call you?

THERAPIST: What would you like to call me?

PATIENT: Oh, so this is one of those shrink tricks where you answer a question with another question? [*Smiling*]

THERAPIST: Oh, so you have had shrinks ask you questions instead of answering yours? [*Patient and therapist laugh together for about 30 seconds, stop, and then resume laughing for another 15 or so seconds.*]

THERAPIST: Seriously, call me what you like.

PATIENT: Anything at all?

THERAPIST: Testing my limits so quick? [*Smiling*] Nothing vulgar, please.

PATIENT: Well, "Dr. Norcross" sounds too official. "Dr. John" sounds like you're my pediatrician.

THERAPIST: Anything in between those sound right to you?

PATIENT: "Norcross," just "Norcross."

THERAPIST: Sure, that works.

PATIENT: And thanks for not being an asshole about it. At the hospital, they were all about rules and titles. Feels here that I can talk freely, and you, kinda, treat me like a person.

That interaction set the tone for the personalized psychotherapy. The client would frequently have new names for me, depending on the content of the last session and his experiences in the subsequent week. Sometimes I was called "Splinter" (the master of the Teenage Mutant Ninja Turtles), "Girl Whisperer" (when we talked about how to approach girls), "The Sex Guy" (when we discussed masturbation), "Freud" (when we examined his vivid and repetitive dreams), "Detective McGruff" (the crime dog, when we explored the negative consequences of marijuana on his mood and medication), and others. My name became the patient's personal idiom and object representation of me. When we successfully finished treatment, the client triumphantly declared that he finally decided on the best name for me: "Sensei."

The methods and techniques used in treatment constitute the heart of activity preferences. Questions that clients might be asked to ascertain method preferences include

♦ "Do you have any thoughts on what we could do together to reach your goals?"

♦ "What kinds of therapy or self-help methods have been helpful for you in the past?"

♦ "Do you have any strong preferences about the particular techniques we use to address your problems?"

♦ "Can you say something about what you'd want to do here to make the most of therapy?"

Virtually any clinical method can be adapted to clients' preferences. Consider the method of parent management training, which has a well-established evidence base but has shown some racial and ethnic disparities in outcomes (Lau, 2006; Prochaska & Norcross, 2018). The wide variation in parenting practices and family values across ethnic groups has led many researchers to adapt the treatment to cultural preferences. Some changes lie at the surface, such as including community-relevant examples, modifying pictures to depict ethnically similar families, and respecting cultural values. Other changes are more structural—for example, recruiting in community networks, matching the ethnicity of the clinician to the clientele, and conducting the treatment groups in churches, where more clients desire to receive services. The outcomes of the personalized parent training typically equate to outcomes for the standard versions; however, the cultural adaptation frequently results in marked improvements in client recruitment, satisfaction, and retention (Lau, 2006).

Another example of matching to patients' method preferences stems from the use of the *miracle question*, a characteristic feature of solution-oriented brief therapy (Kayrouz & Hansen, 2020). The patient is asked to consider, during the night when asleep, that a miracle happens and all their problems are solved, just like that. The therapist then prompts something along the lines of "When you wake up the next morning, how are you going to start discovering that the miracle happened? How will you behave differently? What else are you going to notice?" But some patients will resist or reject the miracle question because they do not believe in miracles. In these instances, a quick accommodation in words or metaphors will usually suffice: for instance, "a fresh start, click your fingers, you at your best, pixy dust is spread on you" (Kayrouz & Hansen, 2020). The point is that, with collaboration and creativity, any technique can be individualized to match the client's preferences.

Of course, there is also the question of the preferred topic. Does the client, for example, want to talk about their past relationships or their present ones, their anxieties or their hopes, their work or their personal life?

The clinician's style is broader than particular methods but not so all-encompassing as a treatment preference. It is about the clinician's way of being with the patient: the general manner, stance, or approach. The C-NIP (Chapter 5) primarily assesses these kinds of qualities, such as the patient's preference for more or less therapist direction.

A general style, which covers several items on the C-NIP, is whether a client wants a psychotherapist who *sits forward* or *sits backward*. Think of it, literally, as your position in the chair. Does the client want you to lean into them: challenging, leading, and actively engaged? Or does the client prefer you to lean back, giving them space, time, support, and the opportunity to use therapy in their own way?

Assessing clients' style preferences is likely to merge into an assessment of their methods preferences, and in clinical practice, there is no need to clearly distinguish the two. Questions that clients could be asked about broader style include

♦ "What style or stance do you find most useful in a therapist?"

♦ "What would you most want from me, as a therapist, in our work together?"

♦ "Which therapist styles do you find repugnant or off-putting? Do you strongly prefer for me to be active and leading or to make space for you to take the lead?"

Patients may hold strong preferences about every aspect of their disorder, treatment, and goals. They may express intense likes and dislikes when it comes to defining the problem; for example, is it more helpful for them to understand ADHD as a disorder, an asset, or a neurodevelopmental difference? This has been described as a process of *co-formulation* (Fischer, 1970; McLeod & McLeod, 2016). Here, the psychotherapist collaborates with the client to develop understandings of the client's distress that make most sense to the client. This process may occur towards the start of treatment, but shared understanding may evolve and be adopted, at any point.

For example, I (MC) worked with a young man, Marcel, who had come to therapy to overcome a fear of speaking in public (Cooper, 2009; Cooper & McLeod, 2011). His previous counseling focused on the abuse he suffered as a boy. This was also the focus of the first two sessions in the current therapy, but in the third session, when Marcel was asked how he was finding the therapy, he said that he was uncertain whether he wanted to go into the abuse again: "I can't be bothered with it any more. Is it just going to be there and I have to accept it?" I replied, "I guess part of the question is how much it is related to the problems that you are experiencing at the moment, and that is what we don't really know." We then explored a range of possible understandings for why Marcel might be experiencing his difficulties, which I summarized towards the end of the third session as follows:

> One is that . . . it is about stuff that happened in your past that has made it difficult for you and has inhibited you and made you anxious [*psychodynamic understanding*]. Another one is that it's something that you're just not good at it, and you may as well give up, and it's not that much about your past [*biological explanation*]. I guess there is another one, that you're talking about there. That is about a pattern that you have got into, or a cycle, not so much caused by things in your past, so much as you've started avoiding doing that kind of talking, and because you've avoided doing it, you've built it up as something that is more and more frightening, and actually if you started doing it a bit more you would, as you are saying, that "It's not actually that bad . . . it's bearable" [*behavioral explanation*].

In thinking about those possibilities, Marcel concluded, "It could be a pattern of behavior I've just got into." Based on that co-formulated understanding, therapy turned towards helping Marcel undo this cycle of behavior through confronting his fears: developing practical strategies so that he no longer avoided speaking in public and helping him develop more positive and supportive self-talk in these situations. By the end of 17 sessions, Marcel's fears of public speaking had substantially attenuated.

Many roads lead to Rome; many therapies lead to success. But co-formulated understandings of the patient's distress and SDM of the paths to take increase the probability of getting there efficiently and effectively.

WHEN TO ASSESS

Having looked at how and what to assess in patients' strong likes and dislikes, we now examine *when* to assess client preferences. The short answers, as to most clinical questions, are, "Whenever indicated" and "It depends."

Precontact Assessments

Before initial face-to-face contact, it frequently proves helpful to ask clients about certain treatment and therapist preferences. Assessment at this early stage maximizes the possibility of matching, choice, and alliance effects, as reviewed in Chapter 3. In a telephone conversation, a CBT clinician might ask prospective patients about their treatment preferences to check whether they are compatible with a CBT model or seeking something different. Equally, if contacted by a Black prospective client, a White psychotherapist can ascertain any strong ethnicity preferences and ensure that working together is suited to the client's wants.

Clearly, the more publicly transparent clinicians are about themselves and their scope of practice (for instance, on their websites), the lower the likelihood that such conversations will take place because clients will already be aware of who the psychotherapist is and what they offer (and do not offer). We thus encourage practitioners to make certain information about themselves and their practice publicly available so that prospective clients are more informed and empowered to make treatment choices. Such public transparency is not possible or desirable in all clinical settings, of course, but the mystique and secrecy of psychotherapy are not compatible with SDM and preference accommodation.

Many colleagues and clinics also begin identifying patient preferences in the initial paperwork or life history questionnaires. An exemplar in this regard is the Multimodal Life History Inventory by Arnold and Clifford Lazarus (1998). That questionnaire is completed by the client before the first session, to accelerate the process, and asks what the clients think therapy is all about, how long therapy should last, and what qualities the ideal therapist should possess. (We review other preferences measures in Chapter 5.) Premeeting information sheets can also invite clients to consider their treatment, therapist, and activity preferences for psychotherapy so that they are enabled to articulate any strong preferences at an initial assessment.

Intake or Assessment Sessions

Initial appointments are likely to be the principal time point at which client preferences are assessed. For therapist and treatment preferences, this is essential, as work cannot commence until clients make some decisions about their preferred clinician and desired treatment tack. For activity preferences, too, assessment sessions are a natural time to determine the kind of in-session styles and tasks a patient is looking for. In the latter case, the discussion may be more akin to the beginning of a dialogue: Further discussions about activity preferences are likely to transpire across the course of psychotherapy.

The timing of preference assessment naturally depends upon the length and format of the initial appointments, but we tend to assess toward the end of the interview. Most patients enter the first contact anxiously, wondering what will transpire, what they will be asked, how the professional relates to them, and so on. We wait until patients express their story or narrative of the problem, usually half-rehearsed, and then work with them to identify treatment goals (the where). Then we ask about their treatment, therapist, and activity preferences (the how). That typically occurs toward the end of the first session. In Chapter 6, we explore what to do when we can, and cannot, meet the client's preferences.

Some clinical settings employ a lengthy or multisession initial interview, involving detailed histories, multiple measures, or structured diagnostic interviews. In those cases, we advise that the assessment of preferences occurs in the second meeting. By that time, clients generally feel more comfortable, some rapport has been established, and it feels natural for them to express their desires. But in all cases, we wait until after the treatment goals have been clearly established.

Ongoing Therapy Sessions

When working with within-treatment preferences, the start of a session is often a helpful time to discuss with clients their preferred methods and topics. The end of each session, likewise, provides an opportunity to review how the sessions progressed and whether the client has any preferences regarding future sessions. There are also certain times, within sessions, when it may be useful to assess clients' preferences. Four markers for doing so are when therapy is not progressing well, when there is an alliance rupture, when the clinician does not know what to do, or when the ending of treatment approaches.

When Therapy Is Not Progressing Well

All practitioners experience times when psychotherapy is not progressing as it should. This fact may be evident from objective indicators, such as scores on outcome or session measures, the clinician's intuitive feel, a patient's laments of dissatisfaction, or any combination thereof. A prime, evidence-based corrective is to collect feedback directly from the client (Lambert, 2010; Prescott et al., 2017). Talk with clients about how they feel therapy is going and whether there is anything that they want to change. Attending to their feedback more often than not transforms an unsuccessful case or premature termination into a satisfactory outcome.

When There Is an Alliance Rupture

An *alliance rupture* can be defined as a "tension or breakdown in the collaborative relationship between patient and therapist" (Safran et al., 2002, p. 236). This may involve the client directly confronting the therapist or a more passive process of client withdrawal and disengagement (Safran & Muran, 2000). Often, alliance ruptures emerge because clients and clinicians hold contrasting views on the tasks and goals of treatment, and reassessment of the client's activity preferences may prove essential at this point.

It is not easy to hear from clients what they do not like about our practices. In the initial sessions with Meena, for instance, I (MC) thought that it might be helpful to share my thoughts on how her depression and binge eating evolved, and I continued to share reflections over the following sessions. During Session 3, however, Meena said to me that she felt interrupted by my "insights," and at Session 5, she specifically asked me to "listen more and say less." For me, this was a bruising experience. Nonetheless, I consciously adapted my way of working: intervening less and sticking primarily to close, empathic reflections. As a consequence, the therapeutic relationship improved markedly, and Meena got more of what she wanted out of the treatment. As we said previously, the data are always friendly—in the long run, at least!

When the Clinician Does Not Know What to Do

When uncertain about what is transpiring with a client or how to move the work forward, a clinician's first response is often to consult with a colleague or supervisor. That is entirely appropriate and advisable. But clinicians (and their supervisors) should also consider whether it is advisable to directly consult the patient on their views. For instance, with Gabriella (Chapter 3), I (MC) was unsure whether she would find two-chair work helpful. On the one hand, it might facilitate her going more deeply into her emotions, but on the other hand, she might find such role-playing artificial and exposing. Consultation with a colleague provided a useful opportunity to explore this dilemma, but consultation with Gabriella, herself, gave the most decisive indication of the appropriateness of this method.

When the Ending Approaches

The impending termination of psychotherapy represents a portentous and potentially conflict-ridden time. Discussing with clients how they would like to approach it can be a valuable collaborative endeavor. Gabriella, for example, raised this several sessions from the end of her therapy, expressing that she felt concerned and anxious about the upcoming termination. I (MC) responded to this proactively: "Do you have any thoughts on how it would be good to bring things to a close?" We talked about it, and Gabriella said it was important that, before doing so, she could address other important conflicts in her life. She also wanted to examine how she could access additional opportunities for treatment.

Scheduled Reviews

Many practitioners schedule reviews of psychotherapy progress at regular intervals (e.g., every 3 or 5 weeks), in addition to addressing client concerns in an ongoing manner. Scheduled review can identify different activity preferences and can also touch on treatment and therapist preferences to determine whether any major incompatibilities have emerged. These reviews range from the informal "How are you finding therapy?" to more structured and systematic analyses of key aspects of the psychotherapy. Questions that a clinician might ask include

♦ "How are you finding the methods of therapy here? What are the things that are helpful and not so helpful?"

♦ "Do you believe that what we're talking about is relevant and useful for you? Are there other things that you think it important to focus on?"

♦ "How are we doing as therapist and patient? What do you strongly like, and dislike, about our professional relationship?"

Typically, such reviews would take approximately 10 minutes at the start of a session. The client's feedback can both inform and propel therapy in the future.

WHAT IF . . .

What if a client expresses no strong preferences?

As we have seen, that may be the case, particularly if clients have not had mental health treatment before or if they desire little control in their lives. It may also involve an unassertive interpersonal style or cultural proscription. It may reflect the fact that the client is intent on "getting on" with psychotherapy and does not feel too strongly about how that's done (provided it works). In that case, prolonging a discussion about patient preferences may prove unhelpful and, paradoxically, be against the client's preferences!

In all these instances, we advise feeding back this understanding to the client and discussing their disinclination (without conveying that they should or must have strong preferences). For instance, a therapist might say, "I noticed that you didn't have any strong preferences for therapy at this time. Is that about right?"

What if a patient says that they want both things, like both directive and nondirective?

Clients can hold equal or both preferences. That typically indicates that there is not a strong preference in one direction or the other. Less typically, it means that they need something different at different moments in therapy. A sensitive follow-up question will, in all probability, clarify the patient's meaning. One client explained that he wanted the therapist to be nondirective and afford space and patience when he wept but to be directive and lead at other times.

What if a patient says they want one thing but then starts trying to do another?

That certainly happens. For instance, clients can say that they want to talk about their past, but in sessions, they focus on present experiences and concerns. Clients' preferences change, or clients, despite themselves, veer off from what they know they need to talk about and avoid core conflicts. The solution? Talk to clients about it: Highlight the disparities and see which paths the client wants to travel.

What if I do not want to ask the client explicitly? Isn't it better to trust my intuitive sense of what a client wants?

Probably not. As we said in Chapter 3, clinicians undoubtedly intuit a lot in their work, but research consistently demonstrates that psychotherapists' assumptions about what their clients are experiencing or wanting are frequently incorrect (Cooper, 2008; Walfish et al., 2012). In addition, as we saw in Chapter 3, we can project onto our clients our own preferences for therapy.

What if asking patients about their preferences results in discomfort or confusion?

Such patients tend to fall into one of three categories: dependent or insecure ("But you are the doctor. How would I know what I want?"), those with conventional (paternalistic) expectations about health care professionals ("You tell me what is best, Doc, and I will do it"), and therapy naive or inexperienced ("I do not know yet; this is all new to me").

The latter group can be reassured that it is completely natural and probably expected not to know their strong likes for a new service. Several alternative routes then present themselves. First, remind patients that they are experts on their preferences: "Could you tell me what you like about people in general?" Second, ascertain preliminary preferences by strong dislikes:

"What are a few pet peeves about interpersonal relationships?" Third, agree to ask about their preferences again after a few sessions.

The former groups of patients pose more clinical challenges, as they do in psychotherapy generally. We advise practitioners to treat their clients' interpersonal dependency, insecure attachment, or rigid conventionality regarding treatment preferences as they would all matters. This will assuredly not be the only instance of those interpersonal patterns manifesting in session, only an early instance.

What if I think the patient's choice is wrong, that what they want is not the best thing for them?

Discuss it directly with them. Tell them about your concerns and your perspective. SDM is about dialogue and working together to codetermine the best solutions. The patient has their expertise, but so do you, and bringing that into the dialogue is a key part of making the best decisions together.

What if I don't want to assess client preferences at all? What about my preferences?

This question is usually asked in a sarcastic or petulant tone by high-reactant colleagues. Our response is frequently: Well, then you are reading the wrong book! Of course, we value and honor therapist preferences, too. Psychotherapy should and can fit the professional as well as the patient.

But here's the critical difference: Not assessing and accommodating, when feasible, your patient's strong preferences directly leads to higher dropout, lower satisfaction, and worse treatment outcomes. That's imposing your preferences at the expense of your client. We do not find that clinically or ethically defensible.

IN CLOSING

We expect that, in the future, clinicians will increasingly assess their patient's likes and dislikes for psychotherapy. Identifying strong preferences is a necessary step to accommodating them and producing better outcomes. These assessments will follow the lead of personalized or precision medicine with treatment decisions collaboratively tailored to the individual patient.

The assessment process will, of course, differ across practitioners and settings. The law of individual differences also applies to psychotherapists. But three clinical imperatives endure across the dissimilarities. First, explicitly conduct the assessment, somehow, some way. Second, however performed, give the patient an explanation and an experience of responsiveness. As Wittgenstein would put it, both *say* and *show* that you are individualizing treatment. Third, begin and end the assessment of preferences with a warm and receptive heart toward the other. Set your heart right to codiscover what will probably work and not work for each individual fortunate to receive your good care.

Moments of SDM with clients may be brief, but these exchanges invariably enhance clients' experiences of collaboration, consensus, affirmation, treatment credibility, and positive expectations in psychotherapy. All five of those relationship elements significantly predict and probably contribute to successful treatment (Norcross & Lambert, 2019). Patients commonly say that they feel heard, validated, respected, and treated like a real person by virtue of being invited to consider their treatment preferences, often for the very first time.

5

ASSESSMENT WITH THE COOPER-NORCROSS INVENTORY OF PREFERENCES AND OTHER MEASURES

We cannot safely assume that other people's minds work on the same principles as our own. All too often, others with whom we come in contact do not reason as we reason, or do not value the things we value, or are not interested in what interests us.

—Isabel Briggs Myers

Ayo, a 24-year-old college student of African descent, came to psychotherapy with me (MC) experiencing anxiety, depression, and interpersonal trauma (Swift et al., 2019). At the end of treatment, Ayo said that he had found the Cooper–Norcross Inventory of Preferences (C-NIP), a preference inventory measure detailed in this chapter, to be "very helpful" and explained that "it meant that I got to make the decisions on paper, rather than telling a person." By this, Ayo meant that it was easier for him to be more open and honest on a form rather than in speech because he was less concerned about hurting the other person's feelings. Ayo also said that he valued the C-NIP because "there are a lot of questions, and they're all very specific, which is great because they're things I probably wouldn't have thought of."

https://doi.org/10.1037/0000221-005
Personalizing Psychotherapy: Assessing and Accommodating Patient Preferences, by J. C. Norcross and M. Cooper

Ayo articulated two of the four principal virtues of any standardized measurement. First, measures tend to increase the willingness of respondents to truthfully self-disclose sensitive behaviors (e.g., Gnambs & Kaspar, 2015). Sometimes, writing provides a channel by which more "personal" ideas and feelings can be expressed. Second, measures allow for a more comprehensive assessment. A client, particularly when anxiously meeting a clinician for the first time, may not be that aware of their strong preferences. By contrast, a measure invites them, as Ayo put it, to think about things that they "wouldn't have thought about" otherwise.

In addition to these two advantages, the use of measures allows for a standardized administration, so that the same questions are asked in similar ways across people and situations. This reduces the likelihood that the clinician's own foibles and biases will get in the way of an objective assessment of what the client wants. Finally, standardized measures allow the patient's answers to be compared against representative samples so that scaled scores can be produced (e.g., high, average, low). We can therefore obtain a relative sense of the strength of a client's preferences.

In this chapter, we discuss the use of measures as a means of assessing clients' preferences. Our focus is primarily on the development and use of our own preference tool, the C-NIP, but we consider other measures and their respective strengths and limitations.

DEVELOPMENT OF THE C-NIP

The C-NIP, based in part on the Therapy Personalisation Form (Bowens & Cooper, 2012), is a brief, reliable, and multidimensional measure of patient preferences designed for clinical use either at initial assessment or as part of ongoing therapy (Cooper & Norcross, 2016). It addresses all three types of client preferences identified in the literature: likes and dislikes for therapists, treatments, and within-session activities (see Chapters 1 and 4, this volume). However, the scaled scores primarily focus on the latter, and specifically preferences for the therapist's style. It can also be used in supervision, research, and training.

The measure is free to use, without permission, and is translated into several languages. The latest version of the forms, instruction for use, and an online site for digital completion of the form are available at www.c-nip.net/, and the forms can also be accessed at www.scranton.edu/faculty/norcross/. The C-NIP is displayed in its entirety (sans color) in the Appendix. Note that Version 1.1 is a slight modification of our originally published inventory

(Cooper & Norcross, 2016), with all items now keyed in the same direction to minimize client mis-scoring.

The Instructional Set

The instructions for the C-NIP read: "On each of the items below, please indicate your preferences for how a psychotherapist or counselor should work with you." Participants respond on a 7-point Likert-type scale (3 to 0 to −3) with labels: "3 indicates a strong preference in that direction," "2 indicates a moderate preference in that direction," and "1 indicates a slight preference in that direction." Zero on each scale indicates "No preference."

The first part of the inventory presents clients with the stem "I would like my therapist to . . .," and then 18 items in which they indicate their preferences from 3 (a "strong preference" for one end of the item) to −3 (a "strong preference" for the other end of the item). Examples of items are "Focus on specific goals"–"Not focus on specific goals" and "Focus mainly on my thoughts"–"Focus mainly on my feelings." In the unscored second part of the inventory, patients are presented with 11 open questions regarding preferences about the therapist, activities, and treatment. For instance, clients are asked whether they have strong preferences for medication or psychotherapy, the number of therapy sessions, therapy format/modality, or anything they would particularly dislike.

The Four Scales

Based on principal components analyses, the 18 items are grouped into four scales with cut points for strong preferences in both directions: Therapist Directiveness versus Client Directiveness, Emotional Intensity versus Emotional Reserve, Past Orientation versus Present Orientation, and Warm Support versus Focused Challenge. These key dimensions underlying style preferences, particularly therapist directiveness and therapist support, have emerged in analyses of other client preference measures (presented in the Alternative Measures section of this chapter) but not more than two on any other single measure. As these analyses have been conducted independently, and with separate samples, they provide a triangulated understanding of the foundational dimensions underlying therapy preferences. These two factors, directiveness and support, also map closely onto the "agency" and "communion" dimensions, respectively, of the interpersonal circumplex (e.g., Horowitz et al., 2006; Wiggins, 1979).

The first of these C-NIP scales also converges with research studies on therapist activity and evidence-based therapy adaptations (Cooper & Norcross, 2016). The research evidence demonstrates the effectiveness of adapting the degree of therapist directiveness to patient reactance level. Specifically, clients presenting with high reactance benefit more from self-control methods, minimal therapist directiveness, and paradoxical interventions. By contrast, clients with low reactance benefit more from therapist directiveness and explicit guidance. This robust meta-analytic finding can be expressed as a large effect size (d) of .76 (Edwards et al., 2019).

Psychometric Properties

The C-NIP was normed on both U.S. and U.K. adult populations (Cooper & Norcross, 2016). Hence, it should not be scored with children or non-native English speakers. Of course, the multiple translations of the C-NIP are appropriate for the normed populations.

All of the C-NIP Version 1.1 scales show adequate levels of internal reliability: Therapist Directiveness versus Client Directiveness, $\alpha = .76$; Emotional Intensity versus Emotional Reserve, $\alpha = .81$; Past Orientation versus Present Orientation, $\alpha = .93$; and Warm Support versus Focused Challenge, $\alpha = .74$ (Vermes & Cooper, 2020).

The four scales are largely independent of each other or, in quant speak, "orthogonal." The two minor exceptions to this, with consistent correlations in the small to moderate range, are that respondents who want more therapist directiveness tend to want more focused challenge ($r = .16$–$.34$) and that clients who want more emotional intensity also want more past orientation ($r = .13$–$.28$; Cooper & Norcross, 2016; Cooper, Norcross, et al., 2019; Cooper, van Rijn, et al., 2020).

Clinical Utility

Use of the C-NIP has mounting evidence of client acceptability and satisfaction (Bowens & Cooper, 2012; Cooper et al., 2015). Recently, patients at a university-based clinic rated its helpfulness an average of 4.1 ($SD = 0.9$) on a 1 (*very unhelpful*) to 5 (*very helpful*) scale. In total, almost 80% of patients rated it as "helpful" or "very helpful," with just under 10% rating it as "unhelpful" (and none as "very unhelpful"; Cooper, Di Malta, et al., 2020). This was the highest rating of all measures used at the clinic.

Qualitatively, clients have also described positive experiences of using the C-NIP (Cooper, Di Malta, et al., 2020). One client, for instance, said that it was the most important measure that they used "because it was personalized for me and how our therapy should be and not how therapists generally should be, so I felt that was very useful for her to know." As did Ayo, clients thought that the form helped them to express preferences that they felt unable to communicate directly to their clinicians, and it also allowed for a more comprehensive assessment of their wants—things they might not have thought of. The C-NIP was also described as helping to keep treatment on track "because," as one client put it, "it made sure that the therapy focused on the here-and-now and how to deal with my current issues." In the small minority of clients who did not find the form helpful, it was primarily because they felt unclear about what they wanted from treatment. One client said, "To put it on paper just felt a bit . . . like I was trying to answer something I didn't really know myself."

Psychotherapists have also expressed clinical satisfaction with the form, albeit in an earlier iteration (Bowens & Cooper, 2012). They thought that it was a helpful means of assessing what clients wanted from treatment such that it could be tailored accordingly and served as a valuable source of reflection and learning about their own practices. In addition, therapists related that the measure was empowering for clients and helped to enhance the therapeutic relationship. In terms of limitations, they thought that the form could lead to increased therapist self-criticism and over-molding to clients' wishes.

An easy way for mental health professionals to familiarize themselves with the C-NIP is to complete it for themselves as prospective (or current) clients. Take it on paper or online, then follow the self-explanatory instructions to score and interpret it. Jot down any other strong preferences you might have to the open-ended questions. Perhaps explore your responses with a practice partner, in place of a therapist. That will provide a lived experience of the C-NIP process.

The Usual Caveats

All instruments have their respective limitations, and the C-NIP proves no exception to the rule. Given its development in Western, developed countries, caution is needed when applying it to other cultures. The measure also evidences skewed response distributions on two of the scales. However, this reflects the clinical reality that clients tend to prefer directive and less emotionally intense therapist activities. As with all preference measures, clients may not be able—or willing—to articulate what they want from therapy, and what they articulate may not necessarily prove what is ultimately in their best interests (Cooper & Norcross, 2016).

In ongoing research, we are assessing the predictive validity of the measure and its convergence with other preference measures (discussed in the Alternative Measures section of this chapter). At the same time, remember that the C-NIP has primarily been developed as a means of supporting therapeutic dialogue on patient preferences, rather than as a definitive measure of wants. As such, we accord primary import to the clinical utility of the inventory.

CLINICAL USE OF THE C-NIP

Clients can complete the C-NIP on paper, a computer, a handheld device, or their own phone (www.c-nip.net/). If taken electronically, the site will take clients through a series of questions, automatically score their responses, and produce a brief report of scores. This report serves as the basis for the subsequent dialogue or exploration with the clinician.

The C-NIP can also be quickly completed and easily hand scored. Completion and scoring of the C-NIP typically take less than 5 minutes. Patients are handed the form and asked to circle one response for the 18 items. They are told to ignore, for now, the scoring boxes. Clients also checkmark or circle any of their strong preferences on the open-ended list at the end of the measure. When completed, the clinician scores the four scales and reviews the checked or circled open-ended preferences.

Scoring the C-NIP is straightforward and explained on the inventory itself (in the scoring boxes). Scale scores equal the unweighted sum of each of the items constituting the individual scales. Thus, sum the five items (three items for the past/present orientation scale) constituting each scale. Then determine whether that scale score indicates a strong preference in either direction. Scores marked with a minus should be subtracted from the total. For instance, if a client scores 3, 0, and −2, the total would be 1; if they score −2, −3 and 2, the total would be −3. For each scale, circle in the scoring box whether they have indicated a strong preference (in either direction) or no strong preference.

In each case, a higher score indicates a greater preference for the first term in the scale title. The C-NIP was normed so that approximately a quarter of client scores will fall into a strong preference on one side, another quarter into a strong preference on the other side of the scale, and the remaining one half of scores into the average or no strong preference range. These cutoff scores are presented on the instrument itself to facilitate identification of preferences for clinical purposes. Any score outside the average range is considered a *strong* preference, as it is in the upper or lower quartile of the normative group of adults in the United States and the United Kingdom.

WHEN TO USE THE C-NIP

In Chapter 4, we identified several points in the therapeutic process when preferences can be assessed, and the C-NIP can be employed at each of these: precontact assessments, initial assessment or intake, ongoing therapy sessions, and scheduled reviews (especially when clients are not progressing as expected).

Precontact Assessments

Treatment clinics and group practices commonly conduct screenings by telephone before making initial appointments. They often send advance paperwork, including informed consent statements, health questionnaires, and life histories. During these opening contacts, the C-NIP, or portions thereof, can be administered with a minimum of administrative fuss and a maximum of treatment responsiveness.

The central questions here concentrate on macro treatment and therapist decisions: strong preferences for, say, psychotherapy, medication, or a combination; individual, couple, or group; a particular gender or culture of the clinician; psychodynamic, experiential, or cognitive behavior therapy (CBT). The clinical staff can decide collectively which robust likes and dislikes are of paramount importance for identification. The 18 C-NIP items assessing in-session activities can be administered at the same time or can wait until the particular clinician has been selected by the client or assigned by the clinic.

Several university counseling centers administer the C-NIP to all incoming clients. The checked or circled open-ended prompts (indicating strong preferences) determine in part which staff member receives the client: the psychiatrist or nurse practitioner for medication, the group therapist for those seeking that format, or a female or gay therapist for those expressing a strong affinity for them. The four scales scores are used in part to determine the fit to clinicians' theoretical orientation and interpersonal style. Once clients attend their initial sessions, the clinician can consult the C-NIP scores to further attune the treatment plan. All this is gained in about 5 minutes of patient time before the first appointment.

Intake or Assessment Sessions

As with preference elicitation generally, assessment sessions often present the ideal opportunity to invite patients to complete the C-NIP. We recommend that clients complete the form prior to a free-flowing dialogue about their strong preferences. The C-NIP stimulates client thinking about their preferences and obtains a standardized and relative measure of any strong likes and dislikes—unbiased by the clinician's own positions. Alternatively, the measure could be used subsequent to an unstructured dialogue to consolidate the client's expression of wants and elicit any new preferences.

Here is some wording that might introduce the C-NIP to clients:

♦ "We want counseling to be as personalized as possible to what you want. So, we'd be grateful if you could spend a few minutes completing this questionnaire to tell us what that is."

♦ "Let's determine what works best for you in reaching your goal of _____. Kindly take a few minutes to complete this form to pinpoint your strong preferences for therapy."

♦ "Research demonstrates that psychotherapy is most successful when it is individualized to patient preferences. Here's a brief, efficient way that we can begin that discussion."

Once the C-NIP has been completed and scored, the clinician can review with the patient any strong preferences that emerge, inviting them to further elaborate on their answers. For instance,

♦ "I can see that you've put here a strong preference for therapist direction. Can you elaborate on how you'd like that to be and why that would be important to you?"

♦ "You've indicated that you'd like emotional intensity from your therapist. Please tell me some more about that."

♦ "I can see that you've circled a strong preference for the orientation of the therapy—what specific approach were you looking for?"

As well as focusing on the overall scale scores, the clinician talks through the client's scores on the individual C-NIP items. An example of this comes from my (MC's) work with Ayo, introduced at the start of this chapter. At assessment, Ayo's score on the Patient Health Questionnaire-9 (Spitzer et al., 1999) indicated severe depression, and Ayo reported intense anxiety and sadness since childhood. Ayo also reported a traumatic event in his past, but he declined to say more. Ayo lived with a partner whom he experienced as loving and caring, but he felt that he was "holding back" from his boyfriend and becoming increasingly withdrawn. Ayo had had psychiatric help in the past but had experienced it as impersonal and insensitive, running roughshod over his feelings.

About 50 minutes into the assessment session, after Ayo had talked about his history and difficulties, he was invited to complete the C-NIP. He took about 3 minutes to do so and then handed the form back to me. The dialogue proceeded as follows:

MC: Let's look through this. This is about trying to understand the approach we want to take. You're saying there [score of –2 on Item 1, "Focus on specific goals"], not so much goal focused, and you taking a lead in the therapy [score of –2 on Item 5, "Taking a lead"] . . .

AYO: I prefer questions because of . . . yeah.

MC: It's useful to have questions.

AYO: It's *so, so* useful for me. I find it really hard because I'm really blank a lot of the time. It's prompting, it's probably the easiest way of getting stuff out of me [*laughs*]. It helps me bring things up and remember things. So, yeah, that's great. As many questions as possible.

MC: OK. You're saying here about having some structure to it [score of 2 on Item 2, "Give structure"]. [*Ayo*: Yeah.] Skills and homework [score of 2 on "Teach skills" and "Give homework"]. Homework, yeah?

AYO: I'm fine with that.

MC: So, what you're saying is sometimes your mind goes blank, and it's useful to have . . .

AYO: It is blank a lot of the time, and I find it a lot easier if somebody's prompting me.

MC: That's really good to know. And then, in terms of the emotional stuff, you want to be encouraged to go into your feelings [score of 3 on "Encourage into difficult emotion"].

AYO: Yeah. I'm at a place where I do want to talk about the past, and I'm OK with digging up that stuff now. It's farther enough for it to not be so traumatic to think and talk about it. And I really want to get into that a bit more, so that's fine. And I am, again, blank a lot of the time, so it's probably good [*laughs*] to have emotions drawn out of me.

MC: OK. It sounds like being pushed a bit—obviously not too hard—to talk about some of the feelings from the past and be encouraged to talk about that [total score of 5 on the "Past Orientation–Present Orientation" scale, indicating a strong preference for the former].

AYO: Yeah, yeah, I'm more than happy for that.

MC: That's good [*turns over page*]. On this one about challenge or support [total score of –6 on the "Warm Support–Focused Challenge" scale, indicating a strong preference for the latter], it sounds like you prefer quite challenging—

AYO: Yeah, yeah, yeah.

MC: That's really useful to know, and it's also important that you can say when something feels too challenging [*Ayo:* Mm-hmm] and actually doesn't feel helpful [*Ayo:* yeah, yeah]. And it feels really like, as you were saying, about some of the people you've been seeing, and it's important to know when it's crossing that boundary.

[*Ayo and I then go on to review his responses on the open-ended questions.*]

AYO: In terms of number of sessions, as many as possible [*MC:* Yeah, yeah]. Length: I'm happy for that to be as long as possible. Frequency, um, how often do you do it? Do you do it weekly?

MC: It tends to be weekly.

AYO: Yeah, yeah, weekly's fine.

This example demonstrates that the C-NIP can be used during intake sessions as a flexible tool to guide a dialogue about clients' strong preferences for treatment. The goal is not to use the measure diagnostically or to achieve a fixed and final assessment of their preferences. Rather, it is to stimulate thought and discussion about the best way of helping patients achieve their goals. In this dialogue with Ayo, probably the most important realization, emphasized by him several times, is that he wants to be prompted and challenged to explore his past and emotions. Such holistic understandings of the client's preferences take precedence over specific scores.

Ongoing Therapy Sessions

In addition to or instead of administering the C-NIP during initial sessions, clinicians frequently use it as part of ongoing therapy, especially to take stock and perhaps reorient therapy with patients not progressing as expected toward their treatment goals. That comprises one quarter to one third of all psychotherapy patients (Lambert, 2010). The results of the C-NIP and other feedback measures can highlight discrepancies between the therapist and patient in activity preferences, treatment goals, relationship styles, and more.

One of our psychology postdoctoral residents (Eve) encountered just such a clinical realization recently. She had worked valiantly to schedule her new patient with the center's overbooked nurse practitioner so that he could begin antidepressant medication quickly, as he verbalized in their first session. But by their fifth session—7 weeks and a medication dose increase later—the patient (let's call him Adam) had not experienced any improvement and, in fact, appeared a little worse. Eve administered the C-NIP and discovered that Adam's preference for antidepressant medication was relatively weak, certainly not a "strong preference." He desired quick relief, not so much quick medication. The C-NIP results propelled them into a course of hybrid solution-focused and CBT methods, to Adam's relief and satisfaction. Had Eve administered the measure earlier or had the therapy-naive Adam clarified his desires, the initial mismatch might have been avoided altogether. In any event, the C-NIP put them together on the same page and eventually on the same desired pathway to success.

Scheduled Review Sessions

Scheduled review sessions provide an ideal opportunity to reassess client preferences on the C-NIP and to determine whether those preferences are maintained or have changed along any of the four dimensions. Patients complete the items again, with reference to how they would like future treatment to proceed. Typically, now that the therapy has started, the clinician uses only the four scales and omits the additional therapist and treatment preference items. However, asking the client about additional strong likes or dislikes can provide the client with an opportunity to raise other latent concerns or preferences.

In the case of Ayo, I (MC) strove to accommodate his initial preferences by adopting a relatively active and probing stance. I encouraged Ayo to talk about his "negligent" and "disinterested" father and a romantic relationship that Ayo had in his early 20s, which he had experienced as controlling and damaging. I thought that the early sessions were going well, but Ayo's responses on feedback measures indicated otherwise. On the postsession Session Effectiveness Scale (Elliott, 2000), for instance, Ayo reported making only "a little progress." At his first scheduled review (Session 4), Ayo verbally confirmed that he was "not sure whether [the treatment] had been helpful or not." He said that he "really didn't know" how he felt about the psychotherapy to date. Ayo described a "bubble" around him, which made it "difficult to let others in."

I invited Ayo to complete the C-NIP again. His responses were similar to those at the initial assessment, though he now emphasized more strongly his desire for therapist directiveness (score of 7 on the Therapist Directiveness–Client Directiveness scale). These preferences were explored in the following exchange:

MC: And are there ways that I can be more helpful? I saw in the form [the C-NIP] about wanting structure. Does it feel too unstructured or . . .?

AYO: Slightly too unstructured. I kind of don't know what to talk about. So, prompting's probably good.

The C-NIP feedback reminded me of how much Ayo wanted prompting and questions and also encouraged me to be more directive. This was important for me because, as a clinician primarily schooled in nondirective therapies, I could easily fall back into a more "sitting back" style. I invited Ayo to talk more about his previous, controlling relationship, and when Ayo said that he could not say—"it feels like a security screen coming down in a bank"—I encouraged him to stay with it and to "open things up" if he could. Ayo did so and began to talk about the way that this partner would twist what had happened to Ayo in his past, blaming Ayo. This led me, again adopting a more directive style, to encourage Ayo to express something about that past event. Ayo hesitated but, with persistent encouragement, began to talk about a painful episode of sexual assault in his teenage years.

At the end of this review session, Ayo and I appraised how it had been:

MC: I wanted to ask—you've been really open, and I've been pushing you a bit more. Has that felt OK?

AYO: Yeah . . . yeah . . . I find it easier to talk about, I think, with you pushing me, rather than just being left to speak.

MC: OK. It's really important for me that you can say, "I'm not going to talk about that," "I don't want. . . ." It's important that you feel safe not to.

AYO: Things come out better when coaxed. I just have that sort of brain [*laughs*].

This case encapsulates many of the points raised earlier in this book: (a) the benefits of explicitly assessing clients' preferences; (b) identifying those strong likes and dislikes throughout the ongoing work, not only during the initial assessment; (c) the therapist's frequently fallible "intuitive" sense of how treatment is proceeding; and (d) the significance of privileging the client's experience of treatment progress. Although the clinician's perspective on outcome brings value, the client's viewpoint proves decisive.

It also proves interesting that, in this case example, Ayo's initial preferences became amplified as the work progressed, rather than reversing or taking a different course. A concern sometimes raised by clinicians, in relation to the C-NIP, is that clients' preferences may change once the work commences. For example, clients who want therapist direction and challenge may come to appreciate a more nondirective therapist style. Undoubtedly, this may be the case in certain instances (see, for instance, the example of Lloyd later in this chapter). However, our clinical experience suggests that, as with Ayo, clients' initial strong preferences tend to remain relatively stable over time. Here, a failure to accommodate these preferences does not bring out a response of "Oh, actually, I like how you are working" but, as with Ayo, "C'mon, when are you going to do the thing I asked for?"

Empirical research has confirmed our hunch that C-NIP preferences are relatively consistent over the course of psychotherapy. The temporal correlations of the four C-NIP scales demonstrate moderate to large stability: from assessment to Session 4 and from assessment to Session 10 ($r = .25–.74$; Cooper, Di Malta, et al., 2020). At least in shorter treatment, patients tend to consistently prefer the same therapist styles over time, even though particular topics and goals will evolve.

USING THE C-NIP WITH ROUTINE OUTCOME MONITORING

The health care world has gravitated to *routine outcome monitoring* (ROM) in recent years. This is the result of converging trends in evidence-based practice and the accountability movement and because of its demonstrated effectiveness in enhancing client outcomes. There are at least a dozen ROM or feedback systems, but two have received the most research attention: the Outcome Questionnaire (OQ) System (Lambert et al., 2013; http://www.oqmeasures.com/) and the Partners for Change Outcome Management System (B. L. Duncan & Miller, 2008; Prescott et al., 2017; https://betteroutcomesnow.com/). Both systems (with adult and the related child measures) modestly improve psychotherapy success for all clients and impressively prevent premature termination among clients at risk for treatment failure (Lambert et al., 2019).

ROM or feedback systems assess patients' sense of how they are faring in psychotherapy toward their objectives (the "where" or the goal) but are limited in measuring how they are experiencing the process of psychotherapy (the "how" or the journey). In this respect, preference assessment is a natural complement to ROM, and we frequently conduct them together.

A self-characterized "lion in winter," Lloyd was a 72-year-old White man in ongoing interpersonal psychotherapy for chronic depression and recent losses. He was closing on a successful business career and a lengthy marriage in which he was the unquestioned man in charge. At the end of the 10th session, his repeated OQ scores showed considerable reduction in depression, and he was progressing as well as, and probably better than, most patients with his presenting level of distress.

Lloyd's C-NIP preferences at Session 10 were dramatically different from those at first administration when he had expressed strong likes for (a) client directiveness, (b) emotional reserve, and (c) present orientation. He began treatment with a strong inclination to be in charge of his therapy as well, focusing on his present distress and avoiding archaeological expeditions into his past, without much drama and emotion. Now, with symptom stabilization achieved with 10 sessions, Lloyd flipped the script and strongly sought (a) therapist directiveness and (b) past orientation (with an average score on emotional intensity vs. emotional reserve).

The therapist was understandably surprised and invited Lloyd to elaborate on this dramatic switch. "I have lots of reasons," Lloyd quickly answered and proceeded to tick them off:

> I am doing better with depression, I trust you, and realize now that I should have done this [psychotherapy] decades ago. I want to understand and resolve some of the shit from my past, and you need to take the lead. I don't know how to do that and have avoided it my entire life.

A lower OQ score, an evolving aim of treatment, and a more advanced phase of the work led to starkly different preferences. The C-NIP provided Lloyd the structure and the voice to individualize psychotherapy in concert with the outcome monitoring. Both genres of measures help clients communicate their progress and preferences, periodically alerting the practitioner to the possible need to adjust treatment accordingly.

COMMON CLIENT CONCERNS WITH THE C-NIP

I don't know what I like or dislike yet.

We normalize this sentiment (as explained in the previous chapter), whether voiced in response to the C-NIP or to an open-ended interview. It proves difficult to record preferences when one does not know them! The therapist can prompt the patient to respond in terms of what a good friend would offer or defer administration of the C-NIP, particularly with patients new to psychotherapy. We *invite* clients to complete the measure, rather than *instruct* them to do so.

I want the therapist to do the things at both ends of the dimension.

Then ask the client to circle the middle 0. That's where they indicate an equal preference for both ends of the spectrum, and you can reassure them that that's what you will endeavor to provide.

I do not know what to put for this item.

Therapists can inquire about the item ambiguity or confusion and provide explanation as needed. Sometimes the difficulty pertains to a particular item wording or meaning; other times, it pertains to not knowing what they prefer (see the earlier response).

I still don't know how to respond.

Usually, ask the client to move on to the next item. If an item is missed, then do not score that scale. The scale norms are based on completion of all items for a particular dimension.

How do I score these negative or minus numbers? I have not had algebra in decades.

Remind clients that you will score the measure for them when they complete it.

What I really want, like being understood and accepted, is not on this page.

You can explain to clients that because nearly all clients want to be understood, valued, and not judged, we did not believe it would prove particularly informative to ask those questions. We developed the C-NIP by reviewing the research and asking therapists about practices that they would be willing to vary (Bowens & Cooper, 2012). In other words, we wanted to know which strong patient preferences could make a genuine difference in clinician practices and psychotherapy success.

All my scores are in the average range.

This pattern of scores will occur for approximately a third of the patients completing the C-NIP. We assure them that is indeed normal and suggests that their preferences are balanced and flexible. We also request that they identify any strong preferences from the open-ended questions in the second part of the inventory.

I do not like completing this form.

A relatively rare occurrence but it does happen (with about 10% of clients, as discussed in the Clinical Utility section of this chapter). We suggest that you sensitively inquire about the client's aversion and nonjudgmentally follow their lead. As the chapter's epigraph declares, "We cannot safely assume that other people's minds work on the same principles as our own."

ALTERNATIVE MEASURES

Although our measure, the C-NIP, provides an efficient, effective, and reliable means of assessing client preferences in psychotherapy, a number of other tools are worthy of consideration for this purpose.

Preference Measures

A range of preference measures, similar in basic design to the C-NIP, have been developed over the years. However, these have primarily been developed for research purposes, with limited clinical testing or application.

Psychotherapy Preferences and Experiences Questionnaire (PEX)

The PEX (Sandell et al., 2011) is a 29-item measure that asks respondents to rate, on 6-point Likert-type scales, the extent to which they believe a range of therapist activities, therapist characteristics, and client activities would prove helpful for them. The items are grouped according to five subscales, derived from research on coping styles and overlapping with those on the C-NIP: Outward Orientation (directive and problem-solving therapist activities), Inward Orientation (reflective and insight-oriented activities), Support (encouraging and friendly therapist activities), Catharsis (emotionally expressive activities), and Defensiveness (avoidant and emotionally suppressive client activities). The PEX subscales have satisfactory internal consistency ($\alpha = .78–.86$), with evidence of concurrent validity (Sandell et al., 2011) and predictive validity (Berg et al., 2008).

The PEX has better established psychometric properties than the C-NIP, but it has its limitations as a preference measure. First, despite its title, it is actually a measure of "helpfulness beliefs" or expectations (Sandell et al., 2011)—the extent to which clients expect to be helped by certain activities.

Second, the items on the PEX form a heterogeneous mix of therapist activities, therapist characteristics, and client activities. This means the results may be difficult to interpret and apply in clinical practice. Third, it has not been directly tested and applied in a clinical setting.

Preference for College Counseling Inventory (PCCI)

The 90-item PCCI (Hatchett, 2015a, 2015b) assesses clients' preferences for therapist characteristics, therapist activities, and client activities. It was designed for use in college counseling, but its items are relevant to other psychotherapy settings. The first part asks seven open questions about preferences for particular therapist characteristics, such as therapist gender and sexual orientation. The second part consists of 32 items focused on preferences for therapist characteristics and activities, with three components labeled Therapist Expertise, Therapist Warmth, and Therapist Directiveness. The third part consists of 28 items on preferences for client activities, with two components: Task-oriented Activities and Experiential/Insight-Oriented Activities. Each of the five subscales showed good inter-item reliability ($\alpha = .89–.92$).

Like the PEX, the PCCI has well-established psychometric properties and covers a broad range of preference dimensions. However, at 90 items, it is very long for a clinical tool, and it was developed on and for a nonclinical undergraduate population.

Counseling Preference Form (CPF)

The CPF (Goates-Jones & Hill, 2008) asks clients to select which of 10 therapist activities they would prefer their counselors to use. Five of the therapist activities are labeled "insight skills" (e.g., being helped to gain a new perspective on problems), and five are labeled "action skills" (e.g., being taught specific skills to deal with problems). The CPF is even briefer than the C-NIP but has just two dimensions and limited evidence of reliability and validity. The scoring procedure is also based on the assumption that preferences for insight and action skills are opposing ends of a single dimension.

Session Rating Scale (SRS)

The SRS (Miller et al., 2002) cannot be considered a formal preference measure; however, it is a widely used feedback measure in psychotherapy and generates indications of client satisfaction with current treatment. The SRS is generally used at the end of sessions and asks clients to indicate on four lines (a) how much they felt heard, understood, and respected in that session; (b) how much they worked on what they wanted to; (c) whether the therapist's approach was a good fit for them; and (d) overall how "right" the session was for them. The brevity of the SRS means that it can be used on a session-by-session basis, giving regular feedback on the match between clients' preferences and the psychotherapy. In contrast to the C-NIP, the SRS only indicates broad areas of satisfaction and dissatisfaction. However, the two tools can be used in tandem to identify mismatches and develop a more sensitive understanding of what the client wants and does not want.

Preference Interviews

The Treatment Preference Interview (Vollmer et al., 2009; see Table 5.1) is a semi-structured, discussion-based schedule that assesses a range of client preferences. In the first part of the interview, patients are asked about

TABLE 5.1. Treatment Preference Interview

Preference	Question content and representative examples
Therapist's characteristics	Strong preferences for counselor gender, age, ethnicity or race, language, sexual orientation, religion, or other?
Activity preferences	Prior therapy or experience being helped: What was most helpful? What was the worst a therapist could do?
	Preferences for the counselor's approach: a therapist who takes charge and is active and expressive, or client taking charge and the therapist is more quiet and reserved?
	Preferences for treatment modality: individual, couple, group, or family sessions?
	Preferences for therapy tasks: try new things between sessions, reading self-help books, watching self-help movies, going online?
Type of therapy	Beliefs about the causes of the problem: will of God, unlucky experiences, biological makeup, unmet emotional needs, unrealistic expectations, relationship conflicts, lack of self-knowledge, lifestyle, or lack of will power?
	Preferences for type of therapy: solution-focused, cognitive behavior, or psychodynamic therapy? (Therapy descriptions include typical goals, therapist–client relationship, and tasks.)
	Preferences for who decides the type of therapy: client makes the decision, client and therapist collaborate, or therapist makes the decision?

Note. From "A Therapy Preferences Interview: Empowering Clients by Offering Choices," by B. Vollmer, J. Grote, R. Lange, and C. Walker, 2009, *Psychotherapy Bulletin*, *44*(2), p. 36 (https://societyforpsychotherapy.org/wp-content/uploads/2018/11/2009-Psychotherapy-Bulletin-Volume-44-Number-2.pdf). Copyright 2009 by the Society for the Advancement of Psychotherapy. Adapted with permission.

previous episodes of psychotherapy and what they found helpful or hindering. They are then asked about therapist, modality, and activity preferences, as well as beliefs about the causes of their problems. The final section presents patients with a range of treatment vignettes (see the Preference Vignettes section in this chapter) and asks them to rate their preferences for each approach, as well as whether they would prefer that they, or their clinician, decide on their treatment.

The Treatment Preference Interview, like the C-NIP, allows for a comprehensive assessment of client preferences and may be of particular use for research purposes. Unfortunately, its comprehensiveness is also a liability for clinical use as it is lengthy, typically taking 30 minutes or more. The questions are also limited to treatment choices provided by the developer's own clinic—for example, solution-focused, cognitive behavioral, or psychodynamic therapy. Adapt the alternatives to fit your practice setting.

Decision Aids

Decision aids, or option grids, are a class of health care tools designed to help patients identify and articulate their treatment preferences (The Health Foundation, 2014). These tools provide prospective patients with information about the available treatments for their particular problems. The aids discuss the likely impact and the pros and cons of each intervention. To date, these decision aids have primarily focused on physical health conditions, although they are now broadening out to mental health concerns. They exist both as written pamphlets and as web-based resources (see, for example, https://depressiondecisionaid.mayoclinic.org).

An example of a decision aid in published form is the "i-THRIVE" Grid for low mood in young people outside of state provision (Hayes et al., 2018). This is a 5 × 5 grid, with the five columns giving common forms of support, such as "Counseling" and "Computer-based CBT." The five rows address the most frequently asked questions when making a preference-sensitive decision, such as "What will this involve?" and "How will this help me feel better?" On the reverse of the pamphlet are details of how young people and their parents can access such resources.

Decision aids help patients make informed decisions about the best health treatments among multiple alternatives. Such aids prove useful when no option has a clear advantage in terms of outcome and when each option has benefits and harms that patients value differently. Videos, pamphlets, web-based materials, and other aids make the decision explicit, describe the available alternatives, and explicate the possible benefits and risks.

A Cochrane review of 115 studies, encompassing more than 34,000 patients, found that when patients employed decision aids (compared to not), they improved their knowledge of the options, felt more informed about what mattered most to them, held more accurate expectations of possible benefits and harms, and participated more actively in the final decisions (Stacey et al., 2014). Indeed, decision aids improve communication between practitioners and patients. However, the research and practice to date have been conducted overwhelmingly on biophysical treatments. Currently, mental health decision aids are not widely available, though we fully expect them to be more frequently utilized in behavioral health and addictions in the coming years (Norcross et al., 2017).

Preference Vignettes

Within research studies, a standard method of assessing clients' treatment preferences has been to provide them with written vignettes (e.g., King et al., 2000) or video recordings (e.g., Devine & Fernald, 1973) of different interventions. Clients are then asked to indicate which of these treatments they would prefer or to rate the strength of their preferences. Examples of preference vignettes were presented in Chapter 4 when considering the assessment of treatment preferences.

Clinically, in comparison to the C-NIP, these methods have the advantage of assessing client preferences to full treatment packages, rather than to specific activities. Hence, they are more appropriate than the C-NIP when asking clients to choose between two or more discrete treatments.

However, treatment vignettes in psychotherapy are limited in several ways. First, the vignettes do not identify any preferences for therapist characteristics or, as mentioned previously, any in-session activities. Second, the vignettes require a forced choice among a limited selection of treatment options. Third, the strength of the preference is not typically gauged. Fourth, the amount of evidence that can be presented on any one intervention—whether in written or audiovisual form—is limited such that clients may not fully understand the options offered. Last, evidence that the vignettes can reliably and validly identify clients' treatment preferences is negligible.

HOW TO EXPLORE

Whichever measures clinicians eventually use to assess their patients' likes and dislikes (if any), the subsequent dialogue with clients about identified strong preferences is a vital part of the process. Remember that assessment results comprise only a starting point for a meaningful exchange about how clients can get the most out of their treatment. In the words of Paulo Freire (2018, p. 8), "Dialogue . . . (is) the way by which we achieve significance as human beings." Some examples of how clinicians can deepen the exploratory process follow:

♦ "I can see here that you desire quite an emotionally intense therapy. Can you say more about that?"

♦ "Your responses to the questionnaire indicate that you want me to challenge you. Is that right? What sort of challenge do you think might be helpful?"

♦ "You've said that you are keen to meet every 2 weeks. Do you have a sense of why?"

It may also prove helpful to inquire into the origins of clients' preferences. This typically generates more context and meaning for their treatment desires.

THERAPIST: You indicated here that you strongly seek a client-led approach, one with little structure and no homework. Can you tell me more about where that comes from?

PATIENT: The first therapist I had I really couldn't get with. He had the sessions planned out the moment I walked through the door. I didn't feel like there was much—any—space for me to have input into things.

THERAPIST: So, the key thing is feeling that you can have some say in what is going on. Is that right?

PATIENT: Yes. To be honest, I didn't mind the exercises too much, but it was the way that he did it. I felt like I could have been anyone.

THERAPIST: It sounds like the main issue was about feeling anonymous and the therapy feeling impersonal [*Patient:* Mm] more than the structure, per se [*Patient:* Mm].

No doubt, the practitioner's theoretical orientation and the setting's clinical demands exercise a huge influence on the form that such a dialogue will take. A psychopharmacologist operating in 20-minute medication appointments might establish treatment goals and one or two strong preferences and then prescribe accordingly. A psychodynamic practitioner employed in an open-ended independent practice, however, may opt to let preferences emerge over a number of weeks and carefully inquire into the meaning of each one.

Subsequent chapters in this volume present the ways practitioners can, and cannot, accommodate their patient's treatment preferences. Suffice it to say for now, in this chapter, that exploring and dialoguing about strong likes and dislikes presents a valuable opportunity for clinicians to indicate whether they believe, or do not believe, that they can accommodate those preferences.

It is essential that the therapist does not convey judgment on the client's therapeutic preferences. We learn nothing from summary judgments; we learn from human empathy. Patients should leave the assessment session feeling that their preferences are respected and valued, whatever they indicate.

IN CLOSING

Seasoned therapists will naturally adapt or tailor therapy to individual patients (Kramer & Stiles, 2015), but to do so effectively, therapists must efficiently assess individual patients on characteristics that make an established difference in psychotherapy success (Norcross & Wampold, 2019). Accommodating patient preferences leads the list of transdiagnostic characteristics that make an established difference (Chapter 2). Standardized measures, including the C-NIP, provide a means of making such assessments that empower patients to voice preferences they may not otherwise, in a way that is consistent and comparable across clients. Through stimulating a dialogue on treatment preferences, these tools can develop more tailored treatments, which should better meet the needs of individual clients and lead to improved outcomes and reduced dropout.

6 IMPLEMENTING CLIENT PREFERENCES IN TREATMENT

Everyone can definitely be pleased, but not simultaneously and not by one person or thing.

−Mokokoma Mokhonoana

The quality of health care in the United States and the United Kingdom is exceptional in some categories but dismal in others. Compared with many countries, the United States and the United Kingdom rank poorly in meeting patient preferences and in providing culture-sensitive services (World Health Organization, 2011). In other words, conventional health care has not taken seriously patient culture and preferences.

In Chapters 4 and 5, we looked at how clinicians can invite, assess, and discuss the preferences of each patient. In this chapter, we describe in detail—and illustrate with cases—how practitioners can therapeutically respond to such wants, hopes, and desires. The chapter is organized around the four fundamental choices, affectionately known as the *four As*, about any particular client preference: adopt, adapt, alternative, or another. That

https://doi.org/10.1037/0000221-006
Personalizing Psychotherapy: Assessing and Accommodating Patient Preferences,
by J. C. Norcross and M. Cooper

is, clinicians can *adopt* into the treatment the expressed strong like or dislike, they can establish and work towards an *adapted* version of that strong preference, they can explore with the client clinical *alternatives*, or else they can collaborate with the client on identifying *another*, more suitable treatment resource.

ADOPT

The first choice is by far the most straightforward and pleasant for practitioners: integrating the client's strong preferences into treatment. What's not to like? Patients typically feel respected and heard, practitioners enjoy tailoring to individual differences, and professional research, ethics, and standards support the entire process. That process is accorded multiple names—accommodating, honoring, integrating, implementing—and we shall employ them interchangeably.

We incorporate clients' strong likes (or avoid the strong dislikes) when they are compatible with our clinical expertise, ethical codes, and research evidence (Chapters 2 and 3). Doing so solidifies the therapeutic relationship, enhances the clinician's confidence, maximizes the probability of client success, and halves the possibility of premature termination. In our experience, at least one of the client's strong preferences can be honored in the course of psychotherapy; indeed, we cannot locate a single exception among our patients.

We adopt preferences when the best available research, clinical expertise, and patient preferences—the triumvirate of evidence-based practice—converge, as graphically illustrated in the Venn diagram of Figure 6.1 (based on Norcross et al., 2017). Here, substantial overlap exists; all three sources are largely in agreement on how to proceed in practice. If only all treatment decisions proved so consensual and easy!

Let's consider the assessment and treatment of Annique's recurrent major depression. For reasons of cost and style, her treatment preference was for a time-limited, active psychotherapy with, in her words, a focus on "the important relationships in my life. That's what makes me tick." The research evidence, the clinician's expertise, and Annique's preferences all pointed towards interpersonal psychotherapy (IPT), an evidence-based psychotherapy for treatment of acute depression in which the clinician was trained and skilled.

Here are the strong preferences, gleaned from the Cooper–Norcross Inventory of Preferences (C-NIP) results or in-session questions, from my

FIGURE 6.1. Evidence-Based Practice Components Demonstrating Major Convergence: Adopt

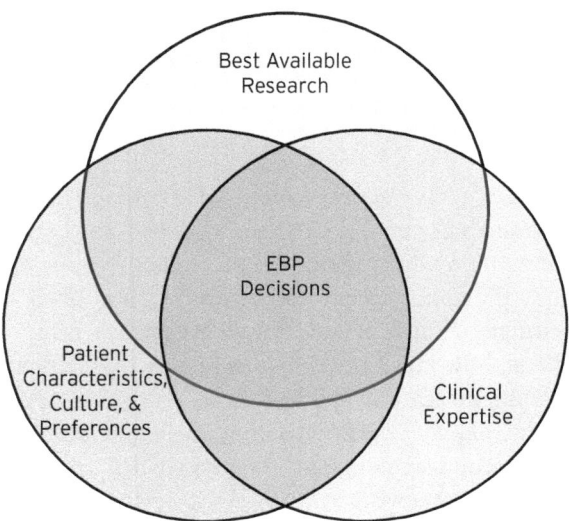

Note. From *Clinician's Guide to Evidence-Based Practices: Behavioral Health and Addictions* (2nd ed.), by J. C. Norcross, T. P. Hogan, G. P. Koocher, and L. A. Maggio, 2017, Oxford University Press (https://doi.org/10.1093/med:psych/9780190621933.001.0001). Copyright 2017 by J. C. Norcross, T. P. Hogan, G. P. Koocher, and L. A. Maggio. Adapted with permission.

(JCN's) last 10 adolescent and adult outpatients. I subsequently adopted all of these activity preferences throughout treatment:

♦ develop between-session exercises or homework assignments ("need to put the talk into action")

♦ refrain from repetitive "uh-huhs" (minimal encouragers) that the client experienced as irritating in a prior therapist

♦ honor ("not judge") the meaning of the client's dreams

♦ combine psychotherapy with an antidepressant medication (prescribed by a colleague)

♦ inform the patient consistently of his diagnosis and treatment rationale

♦ work with the patient's partner in occasional conjoint sessions

♦ recommend some online self-help resources

♦ shun cognitive behavior therapy (CBT; although recommended by her partner) in favor of relational-psychodynamic therapy, which previously proved effective

♦ schedule therapy sessions every 2 weeks in the interest of cost-efficiency

♦ avoid pushing the client into action prematurely: "Let me talk and explore my issues"

Over the years, we have adopted hundreds (perhaps thousands) of the treatment preferences of our child and early adolescent clients. Less verbal and less informed than adults about the process of therapy, they nonetheless highly value the ability to express themselves and exert some control over their treatment. Which person sits where, which game to play, who begins the session, how much the therapist pushes for conflictual material, how to involve parents/caretakers, and more, constitute opportunities for likes and dislikes. Asking youth what they dislike or despise in teachers usually provides a solid working knowledge of what to avoid in sessions, at least initially.

Preference Transitions

Each of the 10 strong preferences, listed previously, was incorporated by me in session and periodically reevaluated for their suitability. In eight of these instances, as with Ayo (Chapter 5), the clients' original likes were maintained because they found them suitable and salubrious. The two other instances, however, were closer to the case of Lloyd (Chapter 5), where the client and psychologist determined that the initial preferences were no longer applicable or efficacious. The seventh session in one of those cases, the last in the previous list, began with the following:

THERAPIST: Usually, I ask you to begin the session, but today, if I may, let me check with you about your strong preference that I not push you quickly or prematurely into action. How have I done? And does that still feel right for you?

PATIENT: Oh, I have been meaning to speak to you about that. I appreciate you asking, and yes, I have not felt rushed into changing my behavior. It's interesting, but I think that is no longer what I need . . . [*trailing off*].

THERAPIST: How so? Can you say what has changed?

PATIENT: Not exactly sure . . . I feel more comfortable here, more ready to make changes.

THERAPIST: When we began meeting, you were unsure and anxious here, and I was a virtual stranger. Also not certain what you wanted to change in yourself. But now, you are more comfortable, more knowledgeable, and, um, prepared to make those leaps. Something like that?

PATIENT: Yes, that's it. All of that.

As is so often the case in practice, it proves virtually impossible to delineate and disentangle what accounts for the transition in preferences. Perhaps it is largely the growth in the working alliance, perhaps comfort with the therapeutic process, perhaps advancement in the phase of treatment, perhaps changes in the client's circumstances, or perhaps progression in the stage of change (from contemplation to action). Client preferences are embedded in readiness to change and the related phase of treatment. As a consequence, the clinical rule of thumb is to accommodate initially the client's strong preferences, examine progress, and reevaluate as necessary. Sometimes preferences remain consistent; sometimes they evolve.

Holding Clients to Task

Sometimes, as discussed previously, clients' strong preferences alter over the course of psychotherapy, and part of the adoption strategy is for clinicians to revise their practices to these emerging wants. From our research and experience, however, we have found that other times clients want us to hold them to their original preferences even if, in the immediate moment, they push in another direction. It is as if clients are asking us to hold them to task, knowing that they are avoiding or deviating from what they know they should work on. Such experiences can prove confusing and conflictual to both patient and practitioner, but time and discussion typically resolve the initial confusion.

Marcella, a White Australian banker in her mid-50s, represents a prime example of this. At assessment, Marcella indicated that she strongly wanted to work on two specific areas: coming to terms with the recent death of her father and finally putting to rest the effects of bullying in her university years. In the first session, Marcella and I (MC) agreed to focus on her father's death, and in Session 2, we began talking through some of the bullying experiences. At the start of Session 3, however, Marcella launched into an animated description of the difficulties she was experiencing in her workplace: the micromanaging boss, the work-shy colleagues, and the unappreciative clients. Marcella seemed desperate to talk through these problems—but was she?

MC: We're about 10 minutes into our session. I wanted to check with you—I'm aware that you've been talking about work issues, and that's something we could carry on talking about. But given the preferences you described when we first met, about focusing on your father and your experiences of bullying—I just wanted to see where you'd rather go with things. What would feel most helpful to focus on for this session?

MARCELLA: Yes, actually, let's get back to processing what happened to me at university. I feel like these work issues are just ongoing.

Subsequent sessions with this client started much the same way: Marcella animatedly talking about some area of her immediate life, then me inviting her to consider whether she wanted to continue with that topic or refocus on what she had initially laid out as her preferred treatment focus. Invariably, Marcella indicated that she wanted to be kept to task and for me to challenge her tendency towards digression. Together, we effectively identified and conquered her avoidance tendencies.

Interestingly, on C-NIP Item 16, which asks whether patients want their therapist to interrupt them and keep them focused, or not interrupt them, we find around 40% of clients opting for interruption, with an additional 20% indicating "No or equal preference" (Cooper et al., 2017). Research has shown, then, that some patients do consciously want to be helped "against" themselves—paradoxically, the client's preference can sometimes be for the clinician to ignore their immediate, short-term preferences! But the only way for the practitioner to know whether this is the case is to discuss it explicitly with clients.

Avoid Going Beyond One's Scope of Practice

Adopting to client preferences should not take clinicians beyond their scope of practice (Chapter 4), but it can take them up to its edges. Managing this balance between authenticity as a practitioner, and being flexible, is one of the essential meta-competencies for preference accommodation. As we saw in the case of Ayo (Chapter 5), the client's desire for prompting and questions led me (MC) to adopt a stance that was more directive than I would typically hold. Yet it was also a therapy style that I felt sufficiently comfortable and competent in: I could draw on aspects of myself—both as a person and as a clinician.

ADAPT

When preferences cannot be adopted, even temporarily, the conflicts are typically with the clinic's or clinician's available resources, clinical wisdom, ethical code, or the research evidence. In many cases, the clinician is not practically able to meet the client's preferences, and alternative options are not available. Offering clients an *adapted* version of what they want has the obvious advantage that it retains as much of the client's original desire as possible and maintains some degree of clinician responsiveness. The disadvantages include the possibility of clients not receiving their preferred approach and thus losing the demonstrated effects of improved outcomes and decreased dropouts. Adapting is a halfway, or three-quarters, measure of balancing these competing considerations.

In adaptation, clients are offered a modified version of their treatment, therapist, or activity preferences when their original preferences seem unlikely to prove effective, and the experienced clinician is highly skeptical as to their worth. For example, the patient expresses an intense desire for a treatment with limited research evidence, such as constantly practicing self-affirmations in front of a mirror. Adhering to that preference will, with a high degree of probability, not serve the client's long-term interest. But ignoring the client's strong desires hurts the therapeutic alliance and treatment outcomes. Thus, we may seek a middle way: a responsive treatment that aligns somewhat with the patient's desires and that possesses proven efficacy.

Those clinical situations are depicted in Figure 6.2. The practitioner's expertise and the best research overlap, but they diverge from the patient's preferences. Indeed, whenever any two of the three circles overlap, but not the third, we typically adapt the client preference. Let us consider three examples, at the level of treatment preferences, of Annique, Jonathon, and Marv, and then another two examples at the level of activity preferences, of Hamza and Jo.

Mismatch: Patient Preference Versus Research and/or Clinical Expertise

In Annique's case, this mismatch would occur when the best research and clinical expertise converge in recommending IPT (or another research-supported

FIGURE 6.2. Evidence-Based Practice Components Demonstrating Major Convergence Between Research Evidence and Clinical Expertise but Minimal Overlap With Patient Preferences: Adapt

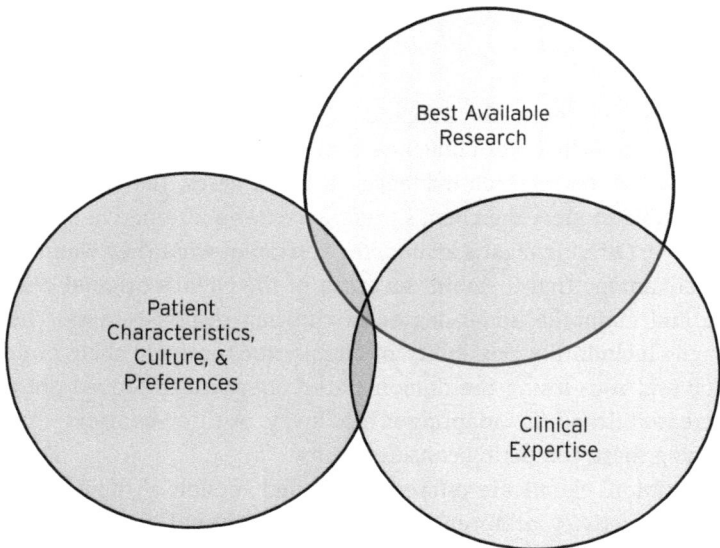

Note. From *Clinician's Guide to Evidence-Based Practices: Behavioral Health and Addictions* (2nd ed.), by J. C. Norcross, T. P. Hogan, G. P. Koocher, and L. A. Maggio, 2017, Oxford University Press (https://doi.org/10.1093/med:psych/9780190621933.001.0001). Copyright 2017 by J. C. Norcross, T. P. Hogan, G. P. Koocher, and L. A. Maggio. Adapted with permission.

therapy) and antidepressant medication to treat her recurrent depression, but Annique rejects one or both of these components. For instance, she might

♦ want to discontinue antidepressant medications due to a dislike of "chemical solutions";

♦ express a preference for a discredited treatment, such as sitting an hour a day in an "orgone energy" accumulator (Norcross et al., 2006); or

♦ decide that her primary goal lies in developing insight into the intrapsychic and family origins of her depression, as opposed to focusing on symptom reduction.

Adaptation would attempt to preserve some of her preferences while maintaining beneficence and an effective treatment. The therapist thus might offer a research-supported insight-oriented therapy, such as brief psychodynamic therapy, without medication for her depression. That adapted treatment plan thus realigns Annique's strong preferences with the best available research and clinical expertise.

Or take the example of a child, Jonathon, an engaging and rambunctious 8-year-old White boy suffering from attention-deficit/hyperactivity disorder (ADHD; mixed type) and mild to moderate oppositional defiant disorder accompanied by family tensions (Norcross et al., 2017). Here, research supports the efficacy of parent management training, stimulant medication, and classroom management for Jonathon's ADHD, and the clinical exper-tise of the practitioner supports all three treatments. Yet, Jonathon's father firmly resists any medication, thus taking it off the table. Both parents are willing to participate in a few family meetings, but their work schedules and marital conflicts prevent extensive outpatient treatment. Jonathon's ele-mentary school teacher already feels overwhelmed by the needs of the other children in her classroom and advocates for medicating Jonathon.

In this case, the therapist adapted the "ideal" treatment plan to accommo-date clinical reality and parental preferences. Medication would not begin until other alternatives were exhausted. Parent management training was offered largely at home by a mobile therapist, which substantially increased its frequency and success. The school principal assigned a teacher's assistant to create and implement a classroom management plan for Jonathon, which improved his classroom performance and attention to some degree, but not sufficiently, so after 2 months, both parents agreed to a trial of stimulant medication during school hours only. Yes, the adaptation entailed more resources, required therapist flexibility and persistence, and delayed its success, but the alternative of insisting on a "take it or leave it" therapist-dictated treat-ment plan would have guaranteed the status quo. The adaptation strategy frequently means taking half or three quarters of a loaf.

Our third example of adapting preferences concerns a delightful elderly patient, Marv, who presented with severe anxiety and depression. He ardently sought individual psychotherapy combined with homeopathic remedies. Alas, homeopathy for mental disorders has been repeatedly shown in randomized controlled trials (RCTs) to be inferior to conventional medica-tions and to produce outcomes essentially similar to placebos (Cucherat et al., 2000; Mathie et al., 2017; Shang et al., 2005). The clinician could have adopted, temporarily at least, the patients' preferences, but Marv's suffer-ing was intense, and he was facing psychiatric hospitalization, which he desperately wanted to avoid. Thus, Marv was immediately encouraged to read several consumer-friendly meta-analyses on the dubious effective-ness of homeopathy for his conditions and asked to consider sequencing his treatment options: first conventional antidepressant medicine for short-term relief, then homeopathy for (possible) long-term effects. He agreed to begin conventional medications as a first step. These quickly reduced his suffering, avoiding hospitalization or deterioration, and psychotherapy commenced with success. As a subsequent step, Marv sought homeopathic remedies, but that proved unsuccessful after four different remedies over a 6-month period. He subsequently returned to maintenance doses of conventional antidepressants and occasional psychotherapy sessions.

In the case of Hamza, a mismatch between what he wanted from treatment and his clinician's evidence-based understanding took place in activity preferences. Hamza presented with high levels of depression and anxiety and was becoming increasingly withdrawn from his college and social environment. The therapist's view, based on an understanding of core behavioral principles, was that Hamza needed to be encouraged to get out and reengage with his world. The more he withdrew, the more anxious and isolated he became. Hamza sensed this pattern, as well. However, he also indicated that, based on a previous episode of CBT, it was unhelpful for him to be told by a therapist, "If you don't do what I'm suggesting, you're not going to get better." He related that it left him feeling guilty, ashamed, and even less confident to go out into the world. The adaptation challenge was to find methods of communicating to Hamza that he could change his behaviors, without implying that he was "bad" or "wrong" if he did not. A delicate balance needed to be struck between helping Hamza own some responsibility and, at the same time, avoiding his strong dislike of feeling blamed.

At the level of activity preferences, evidence from outcome research is frequently less available to guide moment-to-moment practice. Nevertheless, mismatches still occur between the patient's preferences and the clinician's training, beliefs, or values. For instance, a middle-aged African American woman, Jo, sought individual psychotherapy with complaints of clinical depression and marital dissatisfaction. She was a self-described "big hugger" and immediately nominated pre- or postsession hugs as a strong activity preference for her male therapist. He, however, was disinclined to hug patients frequently, as a consequence of his personal style, theoretical orientation, and professional ethics. He collaboratively explored with Jo her preferences and respectfully explained his discomfort, professionally and personally, with physical contact beyond handshakes. In the spirit of collaboration and responsiveness, the therapist instead offered to provide "big verbal hugs" and ongoing support. Jo accepted the compromise, and her treatment proceeded to a fruitful conclusion.

Adapting patient preferences due to the clinician's discomfort enters the murky waters of professional conduct. It is the client's treatment, after all, and ethical codes insist that we privilege client autonomy (Chapter 3). But that is not an absolute value; clinicians are entitled to their own preferences, values, and theories. What happens when the two collide?

Three common clashes concern the relative amount of therapist direction/ structure, the extent of emotional intensity in session, and the relational balance of support and challenge. These dimensions are measured by the C-NIP precisely because they emerge frequently. You may recall, from Chapter 2, that we discovered large differences in the activity preferences of laypersons and mental health professionals on two of the four C-NIP dimensions. That calls for proactive discussion of how the psychotherapy dyad will best work together. Psychotherapists should remain mindful that many patients enter treatment preferring that the clinician is directive—providing structure, offering homework, teaching skills, and focusing on goals—far more than most mental health professionals, themselves, would want. Likewise, clients may not share practitioners' preferences for intense expression of feelings, focus on difficult emotions, and discussion of relationship dynamics. Insight- and emotion-oriented psychotherapists, in particular, may need to explain and frame the clinical rationale for their methods and address any initial mismatches with patient preferences.

Mismatch: Patient Preference and Research Versus Clinical Expertise

In still other cases, clients may be offered an adapted version of their preferred approach because, although their treatment, therapist, or activity preference may be consistent with the research evidence, it conflicts with the practitioner's clinical experiences, theoretical orientations, or ethical codes. Adaptations can entail modifying, supplementing, or sequencing preferences that prove suitable for all involved.

Figure 6.3 displays a case in which the treatment preference and research overlap, but the practitioner's expertise or ethics remains out of sync with both. Two of the circles show considerable overlap with each other but not with the third. Here, the clinical decision is decidedly more complex and challenging.

To continue with our example of Annique, her preferences and the research might both support IPT (or another research-supported treatment, say CBT, short-term psychodynamic therapy, or emotion-focused therapy). However, the practitioner favors Therapy X, which Annique does not prefer and for which no controlled outcome research exists (for acute

FIGURE 6.3. Evidence-Based Practice Components Demonstrating Major Convergence Between Research Evidence and Patient Preferences but Minimal Overlap With Clinical Expertise: Adapt

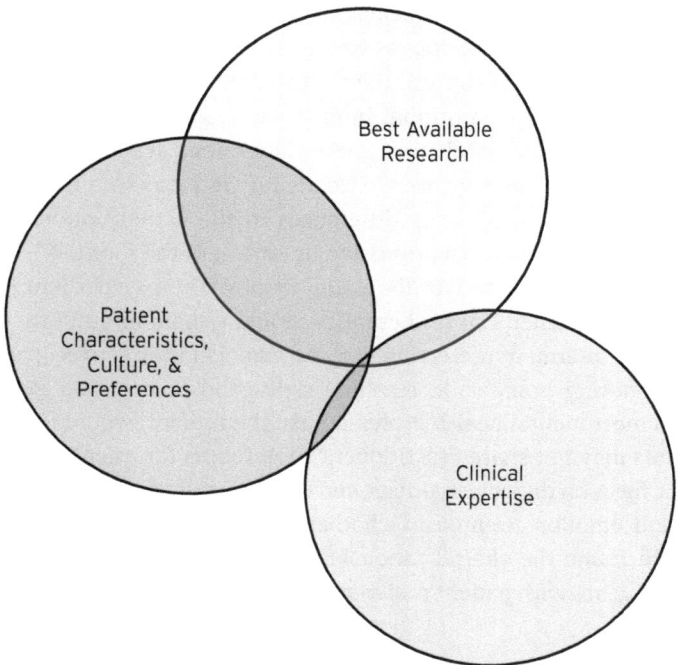

Note. From *Clinician's Guide to Evidence-Based Practices: Behavioral Health and Addictions* (2nd ed.), by J. C. Norcross, T. P. Hogan, G. P. Koocher, and L. A. Maggio, 2017, Oxford University Press (https://doi.org/10.1093/med:psych/9780190621933.001.0001). Copyright 2017 by J. C. Norcross, T. P. Hogan, G. P. Koocher, and L. A. Maggio. Adapted with permission.

or maintenance treatment of depression). The practitioner has skill in rendering diagnoses, conceptualizing cases, forming facilitative relationships, and in other critical areas but lacks both training in IPT and the inclination to obtain it (or, for the sake of illustration, the other research-supported therapies for major depression).

How should the therapist proceed toward a treatment decision? In the face of evidence that IPT works for this disorder, it is not sufficient for the practitioner who prefers Therapy X to rest on the fact that no one has proven it ineffective. One of the research-supported treatments remains the choice and probably the most ethical decision in the majority of such cases. That would result in adopting (not adapting) the patient's strong preference (Norcross et al., 2017).

But in some instances, other factors might mitigate such a weighting and, instead, lead to a decision to adapt. The following are three such factors:

♦ Recent controlled research documents the success of the practitioner's preferred therapy.

♦ In obtaining informed consent, the clinician describes the alternatives and the evidence for each (with decisional equipoise), permitting the client to make an educated decision for their therapy.

♦ The patient has undergone treatment on two or more occasions with the research-supported psychotherapy but has not improved, and now the clinician and client decide that they should elect Therapy X.

The ethics codes of behavioral health professions argue in favor of offering research-supported and patient-preferred treatments, absent such mitigating circumstances. The clinician need not have proficiency in all treatments and may thus refer Annique to an alternative treatment if not trained in that approach (see the next section).

Mismatch: Patient Preference and/or Clinical Expertise Versus Research

Figure 6.4 illustrates a different decision-making scenario: The patient's strong preferences and the clinician's expertise align well, but the best research evidence stands apart. What is the psychotherapist to do: adopt or adapt?

Annique, to continue with our example, presents to psychotherapy with definite preferences for an African American female therapist who will actively engage Annique's larger community, including her church group and pastor, in her psychological treatment. Meta-analyses show that ethnic minority clients definitely tend to prefer ethnically similar therapists over European American therapists (Cabral & Smith, 2011; Soto et al., 2018) but that ethnic minority therapists achieve no better or worse treatment outcomes (Cabral & Smith, 2011; Meyer & Zane, 2013). Hundreds of controlled research studies have investigated the efficacy of family and community interventions, but none, based on our knowledge and literature search, specifically involved church groups in the treatment of depression (Norcross et al., 2017).

Annique's preferences enjoy no support in the controlled research, but neither do we find research literature to contradict them. And the controlled

FIGURE 6.4. Evidence-Based Practice Components Demonstrating Major Convergence Between Clinical Expertise and Patient Preferences and Culture but Minimal Overlap With Available Research: Adopt or Adapt

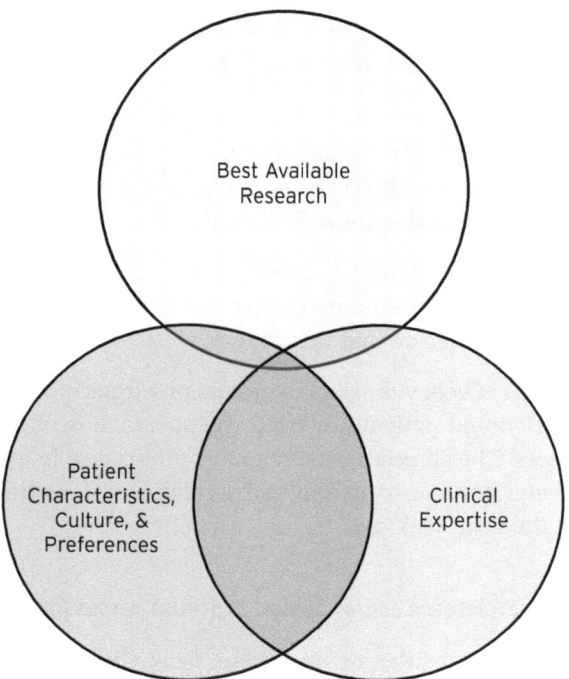

Note. From *Clinician's Guide to Evidence-Based Practices: Behavioral Health and Addictions* (2nd ed.), by J. C. Norcross, T. P. Hogan, G. P. Koocher, and L. A. Maggio, 2017, Oxford University Press (https://doi.org/10.1093/med:psych/9780190621933.001.0001). Copyright 2017 by J. C. Norcross, T. P. Hogan, G. P. Koocher, and L. A. Maggio. Adapted with permission.

research certainly supports accommodating her strong preferences unless fiercely contradicted by other factors (Chapter 2). Annique's strongly preferred therapist, an African American woman, possesses training and competence in working with larger systems, views therapy as a collaborative endeavor, and responds effectively to the patient's values and preferences. She adopts Annique's inclinations, to their mutual satisfaction. Although this particular treatment approach would not appear on a list of "evidence-based" treatments or in a practice guideline, their treatment plan certainly qualifies as "evidence based" in the best sense of that term (Norcross et al., 2017).

In other instances, the decision to adapt would probably be most consistent with professional standards and ethical codes. Sometimes respecting the patient's autonomy and preferences would lead to substandard care. Say that a client repeatedly requested consensually and empirically discredited treatments, as in the case of Marv and homeopathy. We would recommend adapting his strong preferences by adding another more potent treatment, sequencing the discredited therapy later, or educating the patient about the probable (in)efficacy of his preference.

These decisions to adopt versus adapt strong patient preferences constitute some of the most interpersonally passionate and intellectually challenging debates in our clinical careers. How strong are the client preferences versus how strong is the research evidence? Should the clinician honor and trust the patient (adopt) or follow the empirical research (adapt)? Should client autonomy and empowerment triumph (adopt), or should the clinician avoid rendering dubious or even discredited treatments (adapt)? What is the proper balance between respect for patient autonomy and the duty of beneficence?

The pressing point of adaptation is that the practitioner starts where the patient is at and accepts as much of the strong preference that ethics, research, and comfort will permit. That's the thrust of *shared decision making*, a respectful, bidirectional process in which the clinician contributes their expertise. Some dynamic tension occurs in resolving the conflict between adopting wholesale the patient's desire and imposing the practitioner's expertise; however, skillfully done, it is part and parcel of the therapeutic work.

ALTERNATIVE

We respectfully propose *alternatives* to patients' strong likes and dislikes when we believe their preferences will not be most suited to the particular context or when it does not produce the desired results. Before treatment, clinicians may decide that the strong preferences lack applicability and efficacy. During treatment, clinicians may propose an alternative because the patient shows signs of deteriorating, is not making any progress with their preferred approach, refuses to continue it, or threatens to discontinue (Norcross et al., 2017).

Just because a patient desires something does not mean that the therapist automatically provides it. Ethical, legal, and clinical constraints still bind the therapist to responsible and effective practice. In certain cases, the patient may be unconsciously trying to recreate a pathogenic relationship or test the therapy's frame (e.g., McCullough, 2006). In addition, patients may lack *motive congruence*: Their explicit, self-attributed wants and preferences bear little relation to their implicit, actual desires (McClelland et al., 1989). There are indeed limits of meeting client desires.

When unable or unwilling to adopt or adapt patient preferences, we propose therapeutic alternatives. Those alternatives are preceded by, and embedded within, an in-session sequence of processes. We use the mnemonic the *three Es*:

♦ *Explain* your reasoning for not accommodating. This is largely a cognitive frame; for example, ethics do not permit that, or research does not support that preference.

♦ *Empathize* with probable patient disappointment. This is largely an emotional response.

♦ *Educate* patients about the proposed alternative. Conduct role socialization or patient education about the value of, for example, emotional work and in-session discussion of the patient-therapeutic relationship.

Here's a slightly edited and condensed transcript of the male therapist working with the female client who preferred multiple hugs in treatment sessions (introduced earlier in this chapter). He follows the three Es in proposing an alternative.

THERAPIST: I completely understand your desire for lots of hugs in our sessions. That's who you are and how you relate to others.

PATIENT: Yes. My family and I are big on the hugs [*smiling*].

THERAPIST: My code of ethics and, well, my therapy style advises against frequent physical hugs with patients. That's to protect patients, to keep therapy professional. How will that feel to you if we work together?

PATIENT: Not sure. I understand the need to keep things professional, but . . . [*trails off*].

THERAPIST: I sense your hesitancy, you being unsure. And perhaps disappointed that I cannot give you the hugs?

PATIENT: Yes, some disappointment. But I get your reasoning. Hugs can be misinterpreted . . .

THERAPIST: Exactly. And we want no misinterpreting here. This should be a safe place, a trusting place for you.

PATIENT: Uh-huh [*nodding slowly*].

THERAPIST: I would like to propose that instead of physical hugs, I give you lots of verbal hugs—support and validation. That you feel I am embracing you with words. Could that work?

PATIENT: I think so. . . . That's how it works with my [medical] doctor. She's not much of a hugger, but I know that she likes and cares for me.

THERAPIST: That's exactly how I hope you feel about our therapy relationship. Lots of support. And I can certainly meet your other strong preference for homework between sessions. Would you like to try that? Or prefer that we find another therapist who might give physical hugs?

PATIENT: Definitely with you. It'll work just fine.

The relational heart of the matter is listening and seriously considering the patient's perspective. Even when we cannot adopt or adapt the patient preferences, it is done with empathy and validation and full explanation: Share your belief when the expressed preferences are not in the client's best interest so that treatment decisions can still be made collaboratively.

Before treatment commences, there are several areas when we cannot adopt or adapt patient preferences: limits of practitioner competencies, ethical conflicts, and nonprogressing patients (also known as treatment failures). Each of these may merit an alternative approach.

Limits of Practitioner Competencies

Clients may desire a practitioner of a particular demographic (e.g., female, gay, Latinx) or experience (e.g., a therapist who is a parent, married, recovering alcoholic) that does not match their assigned clinician. Or they may seek medication from a nonprescriber or conjoint family therapy from someone not trained or proficient in it.

One of our postdoctoral residents recently evaluated a 21-year-old male client seeking therapy in a university counseling center for social anxiety. The intake interview proceeded well until the clinician described her preferred and well-researched intervention. The client cited religious values that proscribed some of those CBT methods and instead explicitly requested a religious-accommodative approach that entailed trusting God and surrendering to the anxiety, in contrast to cognitive restructuring and exposure. The postdoc had little experience in religious-accommodative approaches and no competence in the surrender or acceptance method but wanted to honor the client's preferences as far as possible. Should the clinician consult a clergy person, try to convince the patient of the value of CBT, begin by adopting the preferred approach, adapt parts of the preference, or propose an alternative?

We were befuddled on how to proceed. Although there is considerable research to support religious accommodation in general (Captari et al., 2018), there are no known RCTs on the client's desired treatment in particular. In fact, most of the outcome research supports the opposite of the patient's preference. We wanted to support the patient's autonomy but simultaneously uphold the ethical principle of beneficence. The bottom-line question was whether the probable outcomes justified incorporating the preference. When we "staffed" the case, fellow clinicians reached no consensus and recommended all of the preceding clinical options.

This and similar case examples can only begin to capture the enormous complexity of combining the best available research with clinical expertise and patient preferences. Risk–benefit analyses and decisional balances are humble paths through the tangled thicket of conflicting considerations. At such moments, we secretly crave the older, discarded practice of mindlessly providing all patients with the identical treatment!

Ethical Conflicts

As in the case of the client who preferred multiple hugs, sometimes clinicians will need to say "no" to a client's wants and offer alternatives because they are inconsistent with the practitioner's ethical or professional frame.

Take the example of a 15-year-old client who had been talking about her suicidal feelings during a counseling session at school. She was furious with her mother, felt let down by her friends, and said she wanted to end it all. Her counselor asked her whether she had specific plans and methods to take her life. She said that she did—she knew where her mother kept her medication. She was thinking that she would swallow it all with a bottle of vodka she kept in her room. The counselor, understandably, was extremely concerned and invited the client to say more about why she was angry with her mother, what her friends had done, and why she had such overwhelming feelings. As the client talked, it became increasingly apparent that, whatever the causes, she was determined to take her life—and was at serious risk of doing so.

"I truly appreciate you being so honest with me," the counselor said, "and I'm sorry you're in such an awful place. It is good that you can share those feelings here." The counselor went on, "And as you know, when we first met, we agreed that if you were at risk of hurting yourself, I would need to let someone at the school know. I would like us to go and talk to your principal and contact your parents straight after the session. I'm not sure how you feel about that, but that's something that we do need to do."

The client balked. "I just want to go home," she said, "I need to get out of here."

The counselor smiled gently but remained firm. It was a situation in which, although she wanted to honor the client's wishes, she needed for ethical reasons to pursue an alternative track. "I do understand that," she said, "and I know how frustrated you feel. But in this situation, I need to prioritize your physical safety. We do need to notify someone."

Eventually, the young client agreed to accompany the therapist and inform a school official, her parents, and her physician. The doctor set up an immediate appointment to see the girl and her parents that afternoon.

Reflecting on this event in consultation, the counselor related that she still felt shaken and uncomfortable by what had transpired: "No one likes to go against a client's wishes," she said, "I hated feeling like I was dragging her to the principal." But the counselor was also clear that she did what she needed to do: Her ethical, professional, and legal responsibility was to pursue an alternative route that assumed precedence over her client's immediate preferences. The fact that she had explained this clearly to the client at the start of treatment—and the client had explicitly consented to this condition—made things easier. In a way, she was holding the client to task: not, perhaps, accommodating her momentary preferences, but working within those that the client had originally recognized was in her best interests.

Nonprogressing Patients

After treatment begins and the strong preferences do not prove applicable or efficacious, the clinician can proceed in many ways. Possible strategies (Norcross et al., 2017) include

♦ determining, in a nonblaming style with the patient, the reasons the current treatment is not working;

♦ revisiting the strong preferences and asking if they had a sufficient chance, or "dose," to work;

♦ returning to clinical expertise and the research evidence to discover other research-supported practices for the particular patient and context;
♦ evaluating the patient's readiness to change or motivational level;
♦ assessing the therapeutic relationship, particularly for ruptures in the therapeutic alliance;
♦ obtaining peer consultation or supervision on the case; and
♦ transferring the patient to another clinician (considered in the next section).

ANOTHER

When a client's preferences prove congruent with the research evidence and best practices, but not the psychotherapist's own competencies, then referral becomes a strong possibility. That ordinarily means recommending another therapist or treatment. The critical difference between offering an *alternative* and proposing *another* is that the former is performed by the same clinician, whereas the latter is conducted by a different person or service.

When Alex, a humanistic psychologist, first spoke on the phone to Jan, he concluded that something did not quite fit. He could not put his finger on it, but he felt almost like he had been talking to a ghost, as if Jan had not been there. She was hidden and opaque. When they met for an initial face-to-face consultation, things became clearer. She described an extensive history of domestic violence. Her husband, recently deceased, had screamed at her, bullied her, and watched her every move in the house. He frequently slapped her as well.

What did Jan want from therapy? Alex asked. Jan replied that she wanted to stop feeling so edgy all the time, feeling the constant sense of threat. She wanted to stop waking in the night, feeling terrified in her bones without knowing why. She wanted the house to feel like her own again, not something that was trying to annihilate her. "I feel him everywhere," she said, "in the walls, watching, waiting." In terms of a particular kind of treatment, Jan said that she had had counseling before when her mother died, and while she found it beneficial to talk and thought the counselor was "a lovely person," it was not what she wanted now. Her doctor had recommended CBT or perhaps "E R something [EMDR, eye-movement and desensitization and reprocessing]," and after hearing more about them, she liked how they sounded. Alex invited her to say more. Jan explained that she wanted something focused, to the point, and direct. "I don't want to talk about my life anymore," she said, "I want to dig my hands into the wall and pull that f***er out."

At this point, Alex recognized that what Jan sought in both treatment methods and therapy goals differed from what he could comfortably and competently provide. He thought his humanistic approach could prove of value to her—particularly in building her insight and self-esteem—but also accepted that this was not what she wanted right now. And her preferences were well supported by the evidence.

ALEX: I appreciate you saying about what you're looking for in therapy, and it's probably different from how I tend to work. But it's great you are able to say about what you want. What I can offer is closer to the kind of counseling you had before.

JAN: Oh, OK.

ALEX: My work is mainly about listening and helping clients talk about whatever they want to talk about. It's open and supportive and encouraging, but I can hear you asking for focus and structure, and it's less of that. It doesn't, for instance, have the techniques that you might have in CBT or EMDR.

JAN: Oh, right. That does sound good. But, yes, I had it before, and it was really good, but, yes, this time, I do think I probably want something more focused.

ALEX: That's fine. Different people want different things, and there's no pressure here to work with me. I've got some colleagues I can put you in touch with who offer what you are looking for.

JAN: So, is that more of a focused approach?

ALEX: Yes. I've got colleagues who do both CBT and EMDR. They are both well-evidenced for the problems you want to address. Shall I tell you a bit about each of them, and we can see which one might sound preferable to you?

JAN: Thanks. I do appreciate that.

As in the case of Jan, before making the referral, inquire into the reasons behind the client's preferences and educate the client, if necessary, on alternative effective interventions. In other words, do not rush to referral: Explore preferences and possibilities, and only when there is a clear mismatch between what the client wants and what the clinician can offer (within the bounds of best evidence) should a referral be made.

There is surprisingly little in the psychotherapy literature on how to successfully refer a client on to another practitioner (though see Cooper &

McLeod, 2011; Leigh, 1998; Walfish & Zimmerman, 2013). The following are principles of referral consistent with personalizing psychotherapy:

♦ Identify what you can and cannot offer clients (your scope of practice, Chapter 4) so that you have a clearer and earlier sense of when referral may be indicated.

♦ Accept your limitations as a clinician to avoid experiencing referral as a sign of personal failure but as your commitment to optimizing care for your clients.

♦ Refer onwards in a collaborative way with the client so that it is experienced as a shared decision, rather than an imposition.

♦ Beware that some clients experience referral as a sign of rejection or their irredeemability, so emphasize that it is due to *your* limitations as a therapist, rather than their failure as a patient.

♦ Have concrete suggestions and specific sources in mind, as opposed to vague referrals to other services.

♦ Obtain proper permission or releases so that you can communicate with the other clinician or clinic; that will ensure continuity of care and play the treatment personalization forward.

PATIENT AND PRACTITIONER DIFFERENCES

As we saw in Chapters 2 and 3, preference accommodation may exert a larger or smaller effect depending on the particular client. Effects tend to be larger in clients with anxiety and depressive disorders, compared with those with psychosis and substance abuse problems (Swift et al., 2019). Practitioners will need to work especially diligently to elicit and incorporate preferences from the latter two groups.

In addition, research suggests that clients who have previous experience of treatment and a higher desire for control benefit more from preference accommodation than those without these characteristics. However, the fact that the magnitude of the effect is the same for clients of differing ages, genders, ethnicities, and years of education suggests that accommodating strong likes and dislikes works equally well for nearly all patients.

We are unaware of any controlled research on the relative frequency or comparable effectiveness of psychotherapists accommodating patient preferences. The only research evidence is indirect, but that research suggests older/more experienced and integrative practitioners probably evince more preference accommodation, which in turn leads to better therapy relationships and lower dropouts. Integrative (or pluralistic) therapies can probably accommodate individual patient preferences more easily than brand-name, monotheoretical treatments. By virtue of greater breadth of relational style and technical methods, integrative therapists will adapt, at least in theory, to the huge variation in patient preferences observed in this study. This may prove one reason that integrative therapy is the most robust in retaining clients; its dropout rate was equal to or better than all other therapy approaches for 11 of 12 disorders examined in a meta-analysis (Swift & Greenberg, 2014).

Clinical experience tends to beget greater flexibility, which likely exerts a small but significant uptick in client outcomes (e.g., Leon et al., 2005; Walsh et al., 2019). Several empirical studies indicate that reliance on one theory and a few techniques may be the product of inexperience or, conversely, that with experience comes diversity and resourcefulness (see reviews by Auerbach & Johnson, 1977; Beutler et al., 1994).

IN CLOSING

We can adopt, adapt, offer alternatives, or suggest another clinician or resource—the four As—in response to our patients' strong preferences. However, as Mokhonoana warned in the epigraph at the beginning of this chapter, everyone will not be pleased simultaneously and not by one person or thing. We must accommodate one patient at a time, and each will desire something different. The vast majority of patient preferences can be readily adopted into treatment, as they converge with the research evidence, ethical standards, and practitioner competencies. But other preferences will conflict—to a greater or lesser extent—with the research, ethics, competence, or practitioner comfort.

In the end, the responsive practitioner performs the integration, or lack of it, with relational skill, clinical flexibility, scientific attitude, and cultural sensitivity while monitoring patient progress and adjusting treatment as needed. Effective and ethical practice requires delicate balancing, recursive decisions, and collaborative relationships to ensure that patients understand the probable costs, risks, and benefits of their—and our—preferences.

7 PATIENT PREFERENCES IN TRAINING AND SUPERVISION

Educating the mind without educating the heart is no education at all.

–Aristotle

In this chapter, we provide a multitude of methods to support professionals in training and other supervisees to assess and accommodate strong preferences. This training will require more explicit ways of honoring those preferences and more systematic ways of educating the heart (in Aristotle's words).

Individualizing mental health treatment to patient preferences has emerged as one of the most valued and popular methods in clinical work among both practitioners and clients. That popularity is difficult to precisely quantify because, to our knowledge, no study has comparatively evaluated their value among representative mental health patients. But there are consistent gleanings from clinical work. One of us (JCN) routinely supervises postdocs and residents (in psychology and psychiatry) and asks them to familiarize themselves with six or seven ways of personalizing therapy (Norcross &

https://doi.org/10.1037/0000221-007
Personalizing Psychotherapy: Assessing and Accommodating Patient Preferences, by J. C. Norcross and M. Cooper

Wampold, 2019). Preferences regularly surface among the top two choices to learn, master, and implement throughout clinical supervision (Norcross & Popple, 2017).

STARTING AT THE BEGINNING

In truth, the goal of routinely honoring patient preferences begins with the selection of students for the mental health professions. That's a few steps back in the training process than ordinary. Programs need to admit applicants who are sufficiently intelligent, of course, but more important, centrally concerned with fellow humans. Relentlessly curious, interpersonally talented, emotionally open, relativistic thinkers committed to individual differences. For these trainees, attending to patient preferences comes easily and quickly. For those enamored with technique and manuals at the expense of the human dimension, not so much. In those instances, as Thoreau (1854) observed in *Walden*, men become the tools of their tools.

Training programs must subsequently structure clinical opportunities so that students work with a variety of patients in diverse settings. With client and location heterogeneity, trainees are likely to gain experience in recognizing and accommodating disparate preferences that a diverse group of clients will hold (Swift et al., 2019). Culturally diverse clients, broadly conceived, will ensure ample opportunities for cultural adaptations and preference accommodations (Bernal & Domenech Rodríguez, 2012). When we encounter trainees near graduation who have never encountered, say, a devoutly religious patient who asks the therapist to pray together in session or an elderly client who demurs at shared decision making, we lament the breadth of their clinical experience. We all must immerse ourselves in the marvelous diversity of human experience.

CULTIVATING COMPETENCIES

Given the salubrious impact of preference accommodation on premature termination and treatment outcomes, supervisors can help students develop competencies in this area. These cognitive, affective, and behavioral competencies include, inter alia, embedding shared decision making and patient preferences within the profession's ethical codes and evidence-based practices (EBPs). Remind students of their profession's ethics on client autonomy and collaboration as well as their profession's statement on EBP requiring incorporation of patient characteristics, culture, and preferences into all treatment decisions (Chapter 3). Trainees will immediately grasp that preferences are not a clinical option or add-on but a professional and ethical responsibility.

Key competencies include

♦ **Understanding the research evidence in support of assessing patients' strong preferences.** Assigning any of the recent meta-analyses or Chapter 2 of this book should do the trick (e.g., Lindhiem et al., 2014; McHugh et al., 2013; Swift et al., 2019; Windle et al., 2019). The research is strong and compelling fodder.

♦ **Learning their own treatment preferences and not unwittingly imposing them onto clients.** We request that our trainees complete and score the Cooper–Norcross Inventory of Preferences (C-NIP) themselves to identify their strong preferences. We then discuss how their preferences differ or do not differ from most clients. Otherwise, they are at risk for projecting their likes (and dislikes) onto patients.

♦ **Identifying their scopes of practice for which services they are (a) competent and (b) willing to offer.** As explained in Chapter 4, this is a lifelong process, and clinical experience typically begets expansion of both competence and openness. But trainees need to start the process early in their careers.

♦ **Creating an in-session environment in which patients are free to express themselves and their dislikes.** This was our repeated take-home in the assessment chapters (Chapters 4 and 5, this volume): cultivating a genuine desire to codiscover and honor individual differences. Setting your heart right, in addition, entails inquiring what patients strongly dislike or despise, which is the final item on the C-NIP.

♦ **Practicing the assessment of strong patient preferences via the clinical interview and standardized measures.** Actively invite clients to express their opinions regarding their preferred in-session activities, therapist characteristics, and treatment formats. We encourage competency-based training in acquiring these new skills; for example, read about it, observe experts performing the skill, deconstruct the skills into separate behaviors, practice it (in role-plays), receive feedback (from peers and coaches), and do it in vivo as the opportunity arises. Practice with and without the C-NIP, until meeting a predefined level of skill.

♦ **Adding patient preferences into care formulations and treatment planning.** Yes, there is undoubtedly an avalanche of factors to be considered in arriving at a treatment plan, but what the client wants must assume import in the decision-making process. Whose therapy is it, anyway?

♦ **Adopting clients' strong preferences into treatment.** This competency poses the most challenges in training. It is relatively easy to embrace "a new therapy for each patient" in theory, but actually changing the therapist's habitual style in the office can prove demanding. We employ variants of *deliberate practice*, a research-supported model to improve student performance and obtain better results (Miller et al., 2019; Rousmaniere et al., 2017).

♦ **Rehearsing in-session discussions with clients when their strong preferences need to be adapted or alternatives proposed.** We neglected this competency in our early training workshops; we implore others not to repeat our mistake. It takes enormous skill, clinical confidence, and emotional regulation to plunge headlong into a discussion of *not* providing what another ardently seeks in a professional relationship. For training purposes, we use the skill modules of *repairing alliance ruptures*, which has been shown to associate with and predict positive outcomes (Eubanks et al., 2018). The requisite steps encompass acknowledging the rupture openly and nondefensively, inviting patients to explore their experience of not receiving their strongly preferred service, empathizing with patients' disappointment or other negative feelings about the situation, validating them for broaching a difficult and potentially divisive topic in the session and not blaming them for misunderstanding or failing to comply with the therapist's wishes.

♦ **Developing the capacity to effectively and nondefensively negotiate referral to another professional.** As discussed in Chapter 6, referral to another mental health worker or organization is a core skill often lacking in training programs. These conversations need to result in patients walking away feeling that they have been cared for and the professional is prioritizing their health.

We and others (Swift et al., 2019) also recommend training students to develop higher order *meta-competencies* in the area of preference accommodation. These include the trainee's capacity to respond to clients when their preferences may be more difficult to accommodate, balance preference accommodation against a psychologically informed assessment of what the client needs, be flexible while also authentic as a practitioner, and recognize the individual client's preferences regarding the treatment decision-making process.

Two final guidelines about cultivating competencies: First, preference training should be formally programmed into a training syllabus rather than scheduled on an informal or ad hoc basis. We have visited and consulted with numerous training programs in which the faculty assumed that such work was being informally performed by colleagues, although it was not being done at all. Second, we reiterate that these competencies should be behaviorally demonstrated by students, not merely discussed by trainers.

PROMOTING EVIDENCE-BASED TEACHING OF AN EBP

Moving research evidence from science to service, from the (lab) bench to the bedside, poses a thorny problem for EBPs across all of health care (Norcross et al., 2017). The gulf between discovery of a research-supported practice, such as preference accommodation, and its implementation has been characterized as "the valley of death," "a clogged pipeline," and the "research–practice gap." Translation(al) research inclusively refers to the process of successfully moving research-supported discoveries into established practice and policy. As a celebrated quote from Göethe puts it, "Knowing is not enough; we must apply. Willing is not enough; we must do."

Supporting trainees to assess and incorporate client preferences in daily practice consists of three distinct but overlapping steps. The first step involves *dissemination*, which entails raising awareness of preference resources and their availability, particularly the supporting research evidence. The second step entails *teaching* the requisite core EBP skills to competence. Trainees need to know how to personalize. And the third step requires *implementation*, which involves getting evidence routinely used in practice. In this chapter, we concentrate on the teaching and training step; Chapter 9 tackles the implementation step.

Researchers have painstakingly reviewed the thousands of empirical studies on effective teaching in higher education. They converge on several best practices (Chickering & Gamson, 1987):

- encourage contacts between trainees and faculty
- develop reciprocity and cooperation among trainees
- use active learning techniques
- give prompt feedback
- emphasize time on task
- communicate high expectations
- respect diverse talents and ways of learning

Please note the conspicuous absence of several time-honored traditions in education: the extended lecture, the moral exhortation (without skill building), the single bullet or teaching method, and the busywork (without impact or practicality).

The research evidence (Norcross et al., 2017) indicates that we can best teach each EBP skill by

♦ emphasizing the practice of new skills;

♦ separating omnibus treatments into separate components or principles;

♦ using supervisor feedback on practice to teach the finer points;

♦ employing both positive and negative teaching examples;

♦ helping trainees integrate thinking and doing during practice sessions (didactic training tends to be linear, whereas practice tends to be multi-dimensional and dynamic);

♦ providing guidance on the boundaries of using the practice, describing when it may be useful and when it may not be useful;

♦ addressing cultural adaptations;

♦ requiring a minimal level of demonstrated competency in each skill;

♦ modeling and role-playing more with less discussion (more practice, less preaching); and

♦ encouraging flexible use of the method (within fidelity).

Our experience and research suggest that online training may prove just as effective as in-person workshops in promoting the use of EBPs. Several studies in psychotherapy (e.g., Dimeff et al., 2009; Rakovshik et al., 2016; Stein et al., 2015) and meta-analyses of studies in health care (e.g., Means et al., 2013; Richmond et al., 2017) have demonstrated that, with the same amount of training and follow-up supervision, online training leads to community clinicians' equal knowledge and adoption of an EBP as in the traditional live trainings. Internet-based training enables many more practitioners to conveniently access such training. Note that these studies did not simply provide online education but personal supervision and consultation after the training.

Three final teaching recommendations spring to mind based on our collective experiences (Norcross et al., 2017). First, make preference accommodation practical and immediate by using trainees' real-time cases—historical examples and the teacher's cases hold less relevance and fewer rewards for the learner. Second, capitalize on students' natural curiosity and enthusiasm for helping: Once they realize that we do not expect them to calculate statistics or perform research on preferences, they will more likely become highly engaged. And third, teach with an eye toward lifelong learning. The goal should focus beyond identifying and incorporating preferences a few times during training to inculcate a lifetime commitment.

CONDUCTING INTEGRATIVE OR PLURALISTIC SUPERVISION

Trainees learn psychotherapy primarily through experience and supervision. In large-scale multidisciplinary surveys, clinical supervision is generally rated the second most important contribution to one's professional development, immediately behind direct experience in working with patients (e.g., Henry et al., 1971; Orlinsky & Rønnestad, 2005). Far more than courses and books and theories, hands-on supervision of actual clients constitutes the learning foundation.

The term *integrative or pluralistic supervision* deliberatively denotes two meanings: supervision itself that prizes multiple methods, modalities, and mechanisms tailored to the client and supervision of psychotherapy conducted from an integrative or pluralistic approach. At times, this ambiguity proves confusing, but we believe it serves the higher purpose of underscoring the inherent parallel processes of integrative supervision. The supervisor remains theoretically flexible in systematically tailoring supervision to the individual supervisee, just as that supervisee simultaneously adapts psychotherapy to the individual client. In this respect, the supervision medium becomes much of the message (Norcross & Popple, 2017).

Such supervision strikes us as an optimal frame for bringing client preferences wholeheartedly into clinical work. Although committed to pluralism and integration, we do not insist that our supervisees adopt it for themselves. Most do, but not all. Our intention is not necessarily to produce "card carrying, flag waving" integrative therapists (Beutler et al., 1987). This scenario would simply replace enforced commitment to a single system with enforced conversion to an integrative system, a change that may be more liberating in content but certainly not in process. Rather, our goal is to assist supervisees in thinking and behaving integratively—openly, creatively, and synthetically in accord with the research. An informed pluralism, a critical relativism in supervision will eventually afford us—and our patients—the greatest returns.

Integrative supervision is favorably received by the vast majority of trainees and other supervisees, in part by avoiding their bitter complaints of the two more detrimental styles of supervisors: remote and authoritarian (Allen et al., 1986; Moskowitz & Rupert, 1983; Nelson & Friedlander, 2001). The remote and uncommitted style tends to generate supervisee struggle or extensive anger. In such relationships, supervisees commonly lose trust, feel unsafe, pull back, and remain guarded. Supervisors who demand conformity and punish divergence from the theoretical "party line" jeopardize their supervisory relationship and subvert central tenets of pluralism.

Here, in the interest of parsimony, we offer a handful of principles and methods that can support supervisees in prioritizing strong patient preferences in their practice (Norcross & Popple, 2017).

Practice What You Preach

Elicit repeatedly and respectfully what supervisees desire from their supervision and what they desire in getting there. This begins with contracting for supervision, setting expectations, and constructing agreements (usually written) that continue throughout the duration. We ask such questions as, What did you most dislike or despise about clinical supervision in the past? How do you [the supervisee] best accept feedback? How directive should I be when we meet? What sort of supervisory relationship works well for you? Do you prefer readings, videotapes, or websites for further learning? What do you want from today's supervision meeting? What are your thoughts on how we should conduct evaluation of your performance and of mine as supervisor?

In fact, virtually all the preference types that we described in the clinical realm (Chapter 4) can be transposed to the supervisory one and act as foci for inquiry and shared decision making: the supervision model, supervisor characteristics, and within-supervision activities such as format, methods, and style of the supervisory process.

As in clinical work, we assess supervisees' expressed desires and genuine needs. And, as with patients, we seriously consider supervisees' expressed desires but are not necessarily bound by them. They form the initial basis for our discussions and eventual supervision agreement; in other words, we start where the supervisee is at.

Like the C-NIP, a measure has been developed to assess supervisees' preferences for supervisory style: the Supervision Personalisation Form (Figure 7.1; Wallace & Cooper, 2015). This checklist invites supervisees to indicate on 11 items their preferences for their supervisor's activities. Items include "Offer theoretical input—Not offer theoretical input," "Offer self-disclosure—Not offer self-disclosure," and "Focus on my client issues & experiences—Focus on my issues & experiences."

FIGURE 7.1. Supervision Personalisation Form

On each of the items below, please indicate your preferences for how you would like your supervisor to work with you. Please put a line through the appropriate number along the item, *with 5* indicating a *very strong preference* in that direction, and *1* indicating a *slight preference* in that direction. If you do not know, please leave the item blank.

I would like my supervisor to:

1. Offer theoretical input				No preference					Not offer theoretical input
5	4	3	2	1	0	1	2	3	4	5

2. Focus on my strengths & abilities				No preference					Focus on my problems & difficulties
5	4	3	2	1	0	1	2	3	4	5

3. Focus on the relationship between us				No preference					Not focus on the relationship between us
5	4	3	2	1	0	1	2	3	4	5

4. Provide more structure				No preference					Provide no structure
5	4	3	2	1	0	1	2	3	4	5

5. Focus on my client issues & experiences				No preference					Focus on my issues & experiences
5	4	3	2	1	0	1	2	3	4	5

6. Offer self disclosure				No preference					Not offer self disclosure
5	4	3	2	1	0	1	2	3	4	5

7. Draw on more than one orientation				No preference					Draw on one orientation
5	4	3	2	1	0	1	2	3	4	5

8. Provide active techniques/exercises				No preference					Not provide active techniques/exercises
5	4	3	2	1	0	1	2	3	4	5

9. Provide reading & reflection outside of supervision				No preference					Not provide reading & reflection outside of supervision
5	4	3	2	1	0	1	2	3	4	5

10. Talk more				No preference					Listen more
5	4	3	2	1	0	1	2	3	4	5

11. Directly challenge me				No preference					Not directly challenge me
5	4	3	2	1	0	1	2	3	4	5

Note. From "Development of Supervision Personalisation Forms: A Qualitative Study of the Dimensions Along Which Supervisors' Practices Vary," by K. Wallace and M. Cooper, 2015, *Counselling & Psychotherapy Research*, 15(1) (https://doi.org/10.1002/capr.12001). Copyright 2015 by John Wiley & Sons, Inc. Reprinted with permission.

Model Theoretical and Technical Flexibility

In integrative supervision, we cultivate multiple hypotheses, expect rich differences in perspectives, and promote free exchanges of ideas. Differences need not turn into conflicts. This shift is more than semantically relabeling "conflict" into "differences"; embracing and valuing differences lie at the heart of pluralism. Most differences turn out to be complementary, rather than contradictory, when embedded within a pluralistic frame and when tailored to individual client and supervisee differences (Norcross & Popple, 2017).

The importance of modeling interpersonal responsiveness and informed pluralism cannot be overemphasized. Not unlike our children, our supervisees learn to emulate what we do more closely than what we say (Beutler et al., 1987). But, too often, supervisors teach in the form of value *statements* instead of value *actions*. Supervisors should reliably model the curiosity and flexibility central to psychotherapy success.

A recent article, subtitled "How Responsive Supervisors Train Responsive Psychotherapists" (Friedlander, 2015), beautifully captures the relational and modeling context in which instruction occurs within supervision. The author of that article articulated several practical strategies to help supervisees repair alliance ruptures, those tensions and breaks in the therapy relationship. She convincingly demonstrated that modeling, supervisory alliance, responsiveness, and instruction seamlessly flow in promoting supervisee growth. Although it is possible to separate modeling and instruction and the relationship as conceptual categories, as done here, our experience in supervision holds that they are nearly inseparable in practice and in reality.

Personalize Supervision to the Individual

One of the most appealing (and effective) features of integrative psychotherapy is that an individualized treatment plan can be tailored to each client. The same holds true for integrative or pluralistic supervision: An individualized supervision plan can be formulated for each supervisee on the basis of their preferences and other considerations. Just as we ask our trainees to behave multitheoretically in their clinical work, so too, we match our supervision to their unique needs and clinical strategies.

Integrative supervision will obviously take into account a number of supervisee variables. Although we cannot specify a priori all these possible variables and their permutations, our supervision experience and the research literature (e.g., Holloway & Wampold, 1986; McNeill & Stoltenberg, 2016;

Norcross & Halgin, 1997) suggest that we can improve supervision outcomes by tailoring it to six supervisee characteristics: supervisee preferences, developmental stage, therapy approach, cognitive style or reactance level, cultural identities, and clinical setting (Norcross & Popple, 2017). Strong preferences lead the list, to be sure, but never constitute the sole consideration.

Each supervisee manifests an idiographic style, sometimes characterized as a *personal idiom* (Hogan, 1964), the unique meshing of personality and method. Supervisors who are attuned to these individualized styles of personality can help the supervisee use special attributes to benefit the therapy, obviously within appropriate limits. Supervisors who fail to recognize and appreciate each trainee's personalized approach, however, will likely provoke considerable upset when their style is being unwittingly imposed on the supervisee.

Actively Invite Supervisees to Share Their Preferences

Just as clients often find it difficult to say to mental health professionals what they want or prefer (the deference phenomenon; see Chapter 3), so do supervisees experience the same reticence with supervisors. One study found that over 97% of trainee psychotherapists had failed to disclose at least one thought, feeling, or reaction to their supervisors to date, with an average of approximately eight nondisclosures per supervisee (Ladany et al., 1996). Most commonly, these were negative reactions to the supervisor; for example, "I thought he was an arrogant asshole who had a big blind spot on how to help me in supervision."

Such research shows that supervisors, like psychotherapists, need to create space for supervisees to feel that their preferences and feedback will be valued. Hence, to rephrase what we said about actively inviting clients to share their views (Chapter 4), it is rarely enough to respond empathically and acceptingly when supervisees voice particular preferences. Rather, supervisees should be actively invited to express their strong likes and dislikes—to experience the supervisory process as a co-created activity and shared decision making. The Supervision Personalisation Form (Figure 7.1) is one structured method to do just that.

Teach Supervisees to Implement Preference Skills

The vast majority of students seeking clinical supervision have not received explicit training in assessing and accommodating patient preferences. To be sure, they have heard the therapy clichés—individual differences, whole person psychology, different strokes for different folks, and adapt treatment to the entire person—and although they hope to assess and accommodate patient preferences, they have rarely explicitly done so in a session. To which we irreverently respond with our own clichés, "The road to hell is paved with good intentions" or, alternatively, "Hell is full of good meanings, but heaven is full of good works."

Hope is not an action plan toward better results; instead, we steadfastly teach, practice, and implement the skills to assess and accommodate strong preferences. Methods to do so were covered in the previous section on cultivating competencies, so here we concentrate on several pragmatic matters in supervision:

♦ Practice the assessment of preferences in supervision before the trainee ad-libs it in session.

♦ Help trainees limit the universe of possible preferences to a few strong likes and dislikes.

♦ Teach how to administer and score the C-NIP.

♦ Respond empathically to student struggles in mastering preference accommodation. This helps them learn. Responding judgmentally does not.

♦ Ask trainees to bring diversity considerations and patient preferences into discussion regularly.

♦ Guide trainees in determining when, and how, they should adopt, adapt, offer alternatives, or refer to another.

♦ Teach shared decision making (Charles et al., 2003): Information must be shared across the dyad, who discuss preferences as a precondition to any treatment decision, and then attain consensus on treatment implementation.

Monitor Client Preferences and Supervisee Accommodation Throughout

Without monitoring and feedback, supervisees can exhibit *behavioral drift*, the ubiquitous tendency to revert to their habitual or baseline style. It proves difficult to maintain, for example, an emotionally intense focus in therapy unless that is also the therapist's natural pattern. Vigilance is required.

In fact, we have witnessed dozens of our supervisees reverting to their own treatment preferences, not their clients' preferences, over time, and for good reason. As we saw in Chapter 2, most therapists want less directiveness and more emotional intensity than their clients. As a consequence, therapist projection or overgeneralization can easily occur.

As correctives, we endorse responsiveness adherence checks, ongoing case reformulation, and deliberate practice to maintain preference accommodating with each patient. Encouraging supervisees to conduct periodic check-ins with clients will ordinarily suffice. For instance, the supervisee might say to their patient, "In our second meeting, you expressed a strong liking for emotionally intense sessions. Have we met that?" In supervision itself, discussion can center on whether clients are attaining their goals and their preferences.

Trainees will undoubtedly learn that client preferences evolve over the course of treatment. The limited research on the topic indicates that therapy-experienced clients tend to shift towards more insight-based approaches (Bragesjö et al., 2004; Frövenholt et al., 2007). Trainees will observe temporal patterns in individual patients once a positive alliance is established and once they achieve some initial success. Many patients are willing to go deeper and be more emotionally intense over time. Thus, tracking treatment goals and desires proves vital.

We advise periodic reviews of clients' strong preferences in session to track these developments, just as we regularly review supervisees' preferences and our success in accommodating them every five sessions or so. This results in frequent and bidirectional flow of feedback, which, we would punctuate, enhances the success of both psychotherapy and supervision (Bucky et al., 2010; Lambert et al., 2019).

Return Repeatedly to the Client

"Back to the things themselves" is the shibboleth of phenomenology. For preference work, our axiom is, "Back to the clients themselves." That is, if we want to help a supervisee know whether, for instance, they should use cognitive behavior therapy or emotion-focused therapy with a client, a leaning forward or a leaning back style, then we encourage them to consider consulting the client. Not only talking *about* them but also *with* them.

Of course, there will be times when this will prove contraindicated. It may not be helpful for a client to hear that their clinician is considering a diagnosis of psychosis or borderline personality or that they are examining the benefits and disbenefits of early termination.

But in relatively egalitarian, ethically guided psychotherapy, supervisees should be encouraged wherever possible to take treatment decisions back to their clients. At the very least, explore the advantages and disadvantages of doing so. Hence, commonly heard phrases in our supervision are, "That's a great question—to ask your client," "I wonder where your patient would stand on this issue?" and "What are ways in which you can determine which of these options the client favors?"

As an example, Rami was a student in a diploma course in person-centered counseling (Cooper & McLeod, 2011). He was working with a client at a drug and alcohol service and, after seven sessions, was feeling increasingly exasperated and lost. The client was in his late 40s, had been drinking heavily since his teens, and had been referred to counseling by his physician, who thought that it might help him reduce his alcohol intake and improve the relationship with his estranged wife and sons. Initially, the client reported that sessions with Rami had been constructive. After about Session 4, though, the client started missing sessions; in Session 5, he turned up drunk, and in Sessions 6 and 7, the client arrived 20 minutes late and, although apologetic, did not seem to be interested in the counseling.

When Rami explored this in group supervision, the supervisor raised the question of what the client might want from therapy. "Er . . . I guess he wants to give up drinking," said Rami, "I don't know. I've never actually asked him." The supervision group discussed the matter further, and Rami came to the conclusion that he needed to take this question back to the client.

Rami's client missed the next two appointments but turned up the following week. "It's good to see you here," said Rami, "and I'm also aware of how many sessions you've missed recently. Would it be OK if we spent a bit of time looking at what we are doing here and how you want to use your time with me?"

The client admitted that he was not sure: It was his physician who had told him to go to counseling, and he had done it because he thought it would help. "Help in what way?" asked Rami. "I don't really know," answered the client, "Maybe cut down on my drinking, improve things with my ex." "Are those things that you want to change?" asked Rami. The client was quiet for a few seconds. "I don't really know," he replied. "I definitely want to get on better with my boys, but I'm not sure if I ever want to see my ex again."

Those goal and preference questions proved pivotal. Rami invited the client to talk more about his relationship with his sons, the first time they had done so. At the end of the session, they agreed that they would spend the next few meetings addressing how the client could reestablish a good relationship with them. And he did just that. When in doubt, take it back to the clients themselves.

INTEGRATING THE C-NIP INTO SUPERVISION

One of the benefits of using the C-NIP with clients is that their scores can be brought into supervision to inform discussions about treatment planning and selection. For instance,

SUPERVISEE: I think, with my client, she's finding it hard to connect with her emotions, and a lot of what we do feels fairly abstract. She talks *about* her emotions, but she doesn't talk *from* her emotions.

SUPERVISOR: Mm. Any sense of what might help her connect more emotionally?

SUPERVISEE: I did think about two-chair work. I'm not sure whether she'd go for that or not.

SUPERVISOR: What did she put on her C-NIP about emotional intensity?

SUPERVISEE: [*Checks C-NIP*] Yes, she did indicate a strong preference there.

SUPERVISOR: She's indicating that, at least at the start, that's something she might be up for.

As in this example, C-NIP scores can be used in supervision to support the selection, or avoidance, of particular methods and styles. The C-NIP gives the clinician an indication of where the client is or might be willing to go—even when the client seems to be pushing in another direction. In this respect, it can support the supervisee in holding the client to task (Chapter 6): reminding the client of the work that they wanted to do and why they have engaged with psychotherapy. The previous dialogue, for instance, continues in the same session as follows:

SUPERVISEE: I suggested the chair work, but my client said she didn't like that kind of thing.

SUPERVISOR: OK, that definitely doesn't suit everyone. So, how did the session go?

SUPERVISEE: Yeah, kind of the same, really. She talked about her girlfriend again and how she feels angry, but there was no anger in her voice. She spoke about it in a detached way.

SUPERVISOR: Did you raise her preference for emotional intensity? Also, let's look. [*Supervisor and supervisee consult the client's latest*

C-NIP.] She says here she has a strong preference for focused challenge.

SUPERVISEE: So, would that be about getting her to go more into her emotions?

SUPERVISOR: She is inviting you, asking you to challenge her. But obviously, you can't make her feel something. I think it's about challenging her with the contradiction between what she's wanting and what she's doing: "At the start of our therapy, you said that you had a strong preference for emotional intensity, but you're tending to avoid that and keeping things on a fairly neutral emotional level. Does that make sense?" Maybe say something like that.

The supervisee took this back to the client, and this time they had a franker conversation about how difficult the client found it to connect with her emotions. When the client started to theorize about this (she was a psychologist herself), the supervisee remembered the client's desire to be challenged and encouraged her back to the concrete actuality of her problems. "To be honest," the client said, "I have felt deadened and anesthetized to my emotions for as long as I can remember." After further discussion, supervisee and client agreed that they needed to concentrate on the client's earliest childhood experiences to understand the roots of the client's emotional anesthetization.

CATCHING QUICKSILVER IN SESSION

The following dialogue gives an extended example of working with preferences in supervision (adapted from Norcross & Popple, 2017). The client is a female college student, and the supervisee, Leah, her psychologist, is concerned that she did not concentrate sufficiently on the needs and preferences of her client. I (JCN) am Leah's supervisor, and I assure her that she did gain a respectable amount of information and that the process of assessing preferences (and additional transdiagnostic characteristics) is likely to become more natural—and less of a mental checklist—over time.

SUPERVISOR: We'll stop it there [the video of the supervisee's session with the client].

SUPERVISEE: Yes.

SUPERVISOR: So, what's your sense or appraisal of that [referring to the segment of videotaped therapy]?

SUPERVISEE: Well, I think that I got everything in that I wanted to, but that's also the problem. I wasn't listening to her [the client] enough. I had my own agenda going, like find out about homework, find out about this, find out about that. Instead of saying, "OK, what's happening? Are you OK?" she kept talking about how she wasn't sure. She was so anxious that I should have spent a little more time focusing on her anxiety.

SUPERVISOR: Sometimes when you are preoccupied with meeting your own lists, it's hard to be present.

SUPERVISEE: Yes.

SUPERVISOR: At the same time, you got lots of material from her.

SUPERVISEE: Yes.

SUPERVISOR: You found out that she does want "so-called" homework assignments or between-session assignments. She's also OK with the [lack of] meds as they are now.

SUPERVISEE: Yes, she does not want meds.

SUPERVISOR: Right. Just leave it where it is.

SUPERVISEE: Right . . . I think part of it was that I was feeling like I had to get it all in because we don't have that much more time to meet. [The client was a senior in college, and it was nearing the end of her final semester.] She came in last time in crisis, and this was the second time I was seeing her. I wanted to make sure I was filling her needs and, by doing that and running the checklist [in her mind], I'm afraid that maybe I didn't . . .

SUPERVISOR: Yes. And you will become more fluid after a while—where you balance both getting the most information to tailor treatment and listening closely to her. But the first couple of times, it seems like most of our attention is focused on gathering information.

SUPERVISEE: Yeah.

SUPERVISOR: You did make wonderful links on how it was all going.

SUPERVISEE: OK.

SUPERVISOR: In fact, I wrote down several instances in which you obtained her preferences. She wants to meet every week. And yes, it all feels a little urgent because she comes in crisis and you have, what, possibly 5 more weeks [until the client graduates]?

SUPERVISEE: No, not even . . .

SUPERVISOR: Did you feel more comfortable asking the client for her preferences during the session?

SUPERVISEE: Oh yeah. I felt definitely more comfortable than I have, but I still don't feel like it is fluid enough. Especially when I'm watching it.

SUPERVISOR: [*Nodding in the affirmative*]

SUPERVISEE: I think that it is a little disjointed. I could have paused more, reflected back, and then moved on instead of rushing to obtain the information [for treatment planning].

SUPERVISOR: You feel like you didn't do enough empathic connections . . .

SUPERVISEE: Right.

SUPERVISOR: Well, I found three of them [in the session segment just watched] . . . judging by her body language and her verbal response. When you said, "You seem to be struggling between what you need and what he needs or wants," she immediately said, "Yes, that's exactly it."

SUPERVISEE: [*Nodding*]

SUPERVISOR: Afterwards, she said she would like homework [between sessions] and meeting every week, and you agreed to that. That's another form of empathy and understanding preferences. . . . She wants action [stage], she wants homework, and she wants a therapy session every week.

SUPERVISEE: [*Nodding*] Uh-hum.

SUPERVISOR: That was a lot of information to get in, what, 2 minutes?

SUPERVISEE: Right; it didn't take very long.

SUPERVISOR: So, it was efficient; it was effective. When you're inside your head saying, "Now make sure I ask all the questions I've read about," I understand that you're preoccupied.

SUPERVISEE: OK.

SUPERVISOR: [*Nodding*] In going forward, do you feel comfortable and competent in offering her preferred form of therapy?

SUPERVISEE: I think so, yes.

SUPERVISOR: For the action stage, you mentioned "cognitive behavioral" [referring to the treatment method that the supervisee plans to use with this client].

SUPERVISEE: Right.

SUPERVISOR: And she's comfortable with homework; you gave her several homework suggestions.

SUPERVISEE: [*Nodding*]

SUPERVISOR: Cognitive behavioral therapy and no medications at this point.

SUPERVISEE: And she wants me to be more directive.

SUPERVISOR: Yes.

This extract illustrates a representative slice of integrative supervision in which an advanced trainee gathers strong patient preferences to arrive at a preliminary case formulation and to adapt treatment accordingly. That's a demanding chunk of work to accomplish in such a brief time, like catching quicksilver, but an increasingly prevalent task in an era of time-limited treatments and managed care. Her treatment plan is based, in this instance, on the client's preferences but also a range of other factors such as time parameters (a few more sessions), the patient's diagnoses, and the patient's stage of change. Remember, systematically tailoring psychotherapy to even one of those transdiagnostic characteristics—such as preferences or stages of change—demonstrably improves the efficacy and efficiency of treatment (Chapter 2).

(RE)DISCOVERING THE CENTRALITY OF PREFERENCES AT TERMINATION

Nothing is as compelling or as memorable as supervisees learning, firsthand, the power of preference accommodation. Educational inputs into supervision, such as discussing meta-analytic reviews, pale in comparison to the experience of a supervisee sitting across from a patient and learning that the assessment and incorporation of their likes and dislikes literally saved the therapy.

The following dialogue takes place after Leah (the supervisee in the previous example) had just finished showing a videotape of a termination session with a second, comparatively long-term client. Leah had asked the male client to share with her those things that worked well throughout the course of treatment and those things that the treatment could have done without. The client responded that he was happy that she did not push him to do homework.

SUPERVISOR: You could see his [the client's] pleasure and his gratitude throughout the session. I know you have other upcoming termination sessions in which you will have opportunities to ask what worked and what did not. So, he got a lot of out of the therapy, especially when he talked about if he could go back and look at his freshman self.

SUPERVISEE: And that is so profound for me to hear because it was a struggle early on. There were things that I had said to him, like "It won't always be this way." And he would say, "I want to believe you, but I don't."

SUPERVISOR: Yes [*nodding*].

SUPERVISEE: To hear him say that and validate the things that I thought . . .

SUPERVISOR: Yes. Your eyes get a little moist hearing that, yes?

SUPERVISEE: Yeah. It reminds me why I do what I do, I guess. In a big way.

SUPERVISOR: It is one of those wonderful moments. And you may have missed the immediate connection [to discussing preferences], but he essentially said, "if you hadn't honored my preferences" and heard what he needed, he would have dropped out.

SUPERVISEE: Yep. And that is twofold: One that we [the supervision dyad] had not been meeting yet, so I didn't know to act on his strong preferences for things like doing homework. Another is my inability if clients come in and don't do homework [a goal from a previous session] then I don't push them.

SUPERVISOR: Well, a lot of this matching is done intuitively. And you read in him somehow that pushing him may have violated what he needed and perhaps may have even damaged your relationship.

SUPERVISEE: Yeah.

SUPERVISOR: The impressive research on incorporating preferences when clinically and ethically indicated tells us exactly that. The dropout rate, on average, is one third to one half less when you accommodate patient preferences. He just handed that research back to you.

SUPERVISEE: Yeah.

SUPERVISOR: And dropouts are one of those things that you don't discover until it is too late. But if you had pushed his dislikes, he may have dropped out.

SUPERVISEE: Yes [*nodding*].

In supervision sessions, we try to connect the early session assessment and adaptations of client preferences (and stages of change, culture, etc.) to subsequent therapy outcomes. That integrates the clinical results with the research findings and, of course, frames it all within termination work. In this instance, accommodating the patient's preferences proved decisive to treatment success.

Although Leah was probably responding intuitively to some degree to what her client wanted, asking explicitly for preferences cuts through imprecise intuition, provides direct answers from clients, and solidifies the therapeutic relationship. We are certain that we have lost clients in the past, despite our best intentions, because we did not systematically inquire and privilege their preferences. We were not on the same page.

IN CLOSING

Personalizing psychotherapy and supervision fits the experience, research, and values of mental health professionals but, we ruefully concede, not the worldview of most managed care and administrators (Norcross & Wampold, 2019). Among payers and policy makers, the dominant image of modern psychotherapy is as a standardized mental health treatment. This "treatment" or "medical" model inclines people to define process in terms of method, therapists in terms of technique implementers, treatment in terms of number of contact hours, patients as embodiments of mental disorders, and outcome solely in terms of symptom reduction (Orlinsky, 1989). This biomedical model proves restrictive, inaccurate, and increasingly discredited. The psychotherapy enterprise is far more complex and interactive than the linear "treatment operates on disorders to produce effects."

Our integrative or pluralistic supervision aligns with professional ethics and the tripartite EBP that privileges best available research, clinician expertise, and client characteristics, cultures, and preferences. That model incorporates the relational and educational features of psychotherapy and appreciates the bidirectional process of treatment, one in which the clinician and patient co-create an optimal process and outcome. That is both the explanation and experience of training to which we aspire and to which Aristotle, with his "education of the heart," would approve.

8 LIMITATIONS AND CONTRAINDICATIONS OF PERSONALIZING

The principle goal of education . . . should be creating [people] who are capable of doing new things, not simply repeating what other generations have done.

—Jean Piaget

Given the positive research and clinical experience on the preference effect, it may appear puzzling to devote an entire chapter to the shortcomings and contraindications of personalizing. Quite the contrary. This chapter stands in full alignment and support of customizing therapy to the individual: Sometimes, personalizing should not occur or should occur on client features other than their strong likes.

Devoting a chapter to the limitations of preference accommodation also communicates our heartfelt commitment to transparently addressing the shortcomings and boundaries of any effective clinical practice. Frankly, we wish more authors would do so! Many psychotherapy books read like extended testimonials, and clinical workshops sound like infomercials selling products. We do not intend to join them.

https://doi.org/10.1037/0000221-008
Personalizing Psychotherapy: Assessing and Accommodating Patient Preferences,
by J. C. Norcross and M. Cooper

Expanding on earlier chapters, we examine here the contraindications and limitations of accommodating patient preferences. In truth, the limitations actually involve finding ways to personalize beyond the typical likes and dislikes. These constitute finding paths to creating a new therapy for each patient. Or, in one of our favorite lines, tailor the tailoring.

CONTRAINDICATIONS

For whom might assessing and accommodating preferences prove contraindicated? We have already reviewed research indicating that individuals with limited experience with mental health treatment and with low desire for control are probably the least likely to benefit from these processes (Chapter 3). Consider, in addition, the following patient features.

Diagnosis

Patients suffering from certain mental disorders may not reliably convey their treatment preferences or have a reduced desire to do so (Morán-Sánchez et al., 2019). These include acute psychoses, manic episodes, delirium, and cognitive impairment. Once the acute episodes abate, clinicians can respectfully engage the patient in shared decision making.

Some persistent personality disorders also pose difficulties in gauging what patients genuinely desire or need. Dependent personality patients invariably either defer to the professional or seek high therapist directiveness, and that style will prove more comfortable (and more effective) to them in the short run (Edwards et al., 2019). However, in the long run, therapist direction strengthens the dependent cycle. In these cases, we advise dialoguing explicitly about the trade-offs. We typically adopt clients' initial request for direction and then, as they improve, ask them to gradually assume more direction for their treatment.

Clients with intense emotional or relational vacillation also challenge therapists in negotiating treatment preferences. Those suffering from cyclothymic, rapid cycling bipolar, and borderline personality disorders can present with strong preferences in one session and then negate those in the next. In those cases, the clinician usually defers on assessment and implementation of preferences until a modicum of clinical stability is achieved.

Culture

Patients' cultural backgrounds naturally impact their treatment preferences, including their willingness to voice those preferences. We have discovered that some older, conventionally socialized patients experience discomfort in expressing their strong treatment likes and dislikes. They prefer the paternalistic stance of most physicians and immediately defer to the professional: "I trust that you know best, Doctor" and "Whatever you say, I will do." Explanations about the value of collaborative care and the effectiveness of tailoring therapy typically do not alter their adamancy. We thank them for their trust and reluctantly adopt their request; it is, after all, their therapy.

Likewise, Asian American patients can experience reticence and difficulty in "telling" their mental health professionals how to proceed (Sue et al., 2019). A cultural-congruent reverent and deferential approach to authority requires some adaptation. We frequently inquire whether the patient knows a way that they would be comfortable in expressing strong likes and dislikes. About half the time, with that freedom, the individual can find a way to do so directly in therapy. Common examples are to describe what they would like from a trusted friend or supportive family member, to explain what they like from their primary care physician, or articulate in general terms what they dislike about people.

During a workshop in Japan, I (JCN) brainstormed with colleagues how preferences could be secured without overt requests. Japanese clients felt more comfortable (a) writing a few strong preferences and slipping the paper across the desk and (b) sending a text or e-mail outlining a few preferences for the clinician to read between sessions. Both methods thereby avoid direct face-to-face discussion, which is the typically Western method. Such encounters remind us not only to tailor the tailoring but also to tailor the assessment of tailoring.

Inapplicable

A final contraindication of sorts occurs when treatment preferences are not paramount. This will transpire on occasion when all of the Cooper–Norcross Inventory of Preferences (C-NIP) scores fall in the average range, treatment goals predominate over treatment preferences, or the client cannot nominate strong likes. In these instances, we recommend that therapists offer choices on other clinical options (e.g., timing, sequencing, frequency of sessions) and consider other effective adaptation methods (e.g., culture, stage of change). Whole patient care still operates.

LIMITATIONS

In this chapter and elsewhere in this book, we have articulated the principal limitation of personalizing psychotherapy to treatment preferences, but we reiterate it here for prominence. Just because patients want something doesn't mean you automatically provide it. Ethical and legal constraints operate. Therapists are people too and manifest limits of professional capacity.

Additional limitations, raised in previous chapters, deserve brief reiteration here. The possibility of patients requesting preferences that recreate pathogenic relationships is a persistent risk. In assessing preferences, clients may not be able—or willing—to articulate what they want from treatment. And what they articulate may not necessarily be what is of most therapeutic value to them.

The founder of multimodal therapy, Arnold Lazarus, was fond of repeating that a skilled therapist was like an authentic chameleon, changing colors and hues to match the singular needs of particular patients. But even chameleons don't do plaid!

That raises three related matters that frequently emerge in our clinical workshops and supervision sessions: To what should we personalize? Whose therapy is it? How adept are therapists at adapting their style? We consider each in turn.

To What Should We Personalize?

Psychotherapists rightfully personalize to patients' goals, disorders, preferences, other transdiagnostic features, the clinical setting, in-session moments, and to a lesser extent, their own preferences. Focusing in this volume on a single area—in this case, client preferences—can unfortunately convey the impression that this is the only effective area. We do not intend to degrade the contributions of other effective ways of adapting therapy. Use all that work! At the same time, as reviewed in Chapter 2, responsiveness to clients' strong likes and dislikes emerges in the research as one of the most powerful methods to enhance treatment outcomes and prevent premature terminations.

Whose Therapy Is It?

As to the half-facetious question of whose therapy it is, the obvious answer is that it is the patient's and, to a lesser extent, the psychotherapist's. Treatment is shared, collaborative, and mutual. Accordingly, the ethical and professional mandate is to match to the patient's preferences, secondarily to the clinician's. We rightfully place the welfare of patients first, but the welfare of practitioners counts too. Many of our supervisees drift back to their habitual practices after temporarily customizing to the client.

Who knows best? Most experienced consumers of psychotherapy know what is working and what is not working for them—the inexperienced not so much. Take the example of the ideal length of treatment. What is enough? Reduction in symptoms but still suffering? Virtual elimination of distress? Attainment of self-understanding? New ways of relating to people or well-being? Self-worth and identity? The latter require more extensive and lengthier therapy, and practitioners can certainly share that knowledge and expertise. But only the client can ultimately decide when enough is enough.

Clinicians inform patients of the probable costs, benefits, and trade-offs, enabling informed choices regarding the alternatives. Patients frequently seek professional care because we can see the bigger picture: additional options, complex considerations, unintended consequences, mixed motives, systemic considerations, unconscious sources, and repeated patterns. Our training, experience, and objectivity help us recognize some unwise moves and perhaps some better alternatives (Dockett, 2018). Having highlighted the centrality of patient autonomy, choice, and preferences throughout the book, let us underscore the value of our education and experience. Together, in combination, the patient's preferences and the clinician's expertise provide the optimal path to treatment decisions.

A related concern is the reification and institutionalization of identifying patient preferences. Clinicians have an uncanny knack for turning a relational invitation into a disembodied assessment, and this is as much a risk with preference work as with any other therapeutic practice. As William James famously put it (1909/1987), "It is but the old story, of a useful practice first becoming a method, then a habit, and finally a tyranny" (p. 728). A genuine limitation of routinely assessing and honoring patient preferences is losing the foundational attitude of respect and curiosity, of meeting the new experience: Keep it fresh, filled with wonder.

How Adept Are Therapists at Adapting Their Style?

Last, there are real bounds to the extent to which psychotherapists can adapt their relational style to fit the proclivities and personalities of their patients. Remember, even chameleons do not do plaid. Although the therapist can, with training and experience, learn to relate in a number of different ways, there are limits to our human capacity to modify relationship stances. It may be difficult to change interaction styles from client to client and session to session, assuming one is both aware and in control of one's styles of relating (Lazarus, 1993).

Decades of training experience and research evidence support the assertion that psychotherapists can authentically differ from their preferred or habitual style of relating (Norcross & Wampold, 2019). Effective therapists are capable of more malleability, more flexible repertoires, and "mood transcendence" (Gurman, 1973; Hill et al., 2017; Tracey et al., 2014). Experience as a mental health professional, according to the research, begets heightened attention to the client (less self-preoccupation), an innovative perspective, and more endorsement of an "integrative" orientation predicated on client need (Auerbach & Johnson, 1977; Norcross & Goldfried, 2019). In fact, several research studies have established that therapists can consistently use different treatments in a discriminative fashion. Experienced therapists are able to help clients respond sooner and to provide a smoother course to recovery (Lambert, 2010).

Thus, clinical experience and a modest amount of research attest that practitioners can shift back and forth among different relationship styles within a given case and between different cases. At the same time, we caution therapists that the blending of stances and strategies should never deteriorate into playacting or capricious posturing (Norcross & Wampold, 2019).

BOUNDARIES OF COMPETENCE AND WILLINGNESS

We return, for the last time, to the clinician's scope of practice introduced in Chapter 4. These concern your (a) competence and (b) willingness to treat patients and problems that you regularly encounter. We recommend practice limits and differential referrals.

All mental health professionals must practice within their bounds of training, experience, and competence. Some do not see child patients, some will not see families, some will not conduct neuropsychological evaluations, and some will not prescribe medication. Those limits are relatively easy to identify oneself and explain to patients.

More challenging are therapist preferences on their practice limits or boundaries. Consider the poles of the C-NIP dimensions. Some therapists, by professional training or personal demeanor, will prefer not to be directive, and others will not prefer clients to lead. Some will incline toward emotional intensity, others toward emotional reserve. Should the therapist's strong inclination contrast sharply with a client's strong preference, then tension ensues.

In these circumstances, the clinician can adopt, adapt, or suggest an alternative to that client preference, as discussed in Chapter 6. Adopting requires considerable work on the part of the therapist to counter their own style. Adapting takes less, but still some, work. Or the clinician can use the three

Es and propose an alternative. Should that not meet with the satisfaction of either member of the dyad, another practitioner is indicated.

That referral should be quite precise or what we call *differential*. Similar to making a differential diagnosis, the clinician makes an educated and specific referral to a colleague who routinely conducts that service or expertly provides that style. For example, I (JCN) strongly prefer not to conduct cognitive behavior therapy (CBT) for dental phobias (dentophobia), despite my training and competence in that area. I recognize the centrality of oral health and find the structured treatment effective but incredibly boring. Thus, I refer such patients and problems to CBT colleagues who are comfortable and efficacious in that therapy. Of course, my practice boundary is communicated to clients early on so that they do not waste time and money meeting with me. Other times, patients' strong preferences emerge during the course of therapy, and they may be differentially referred then.

IN CLOSING

"Different strokes for different folks" applies to personalizing as well. We should expect, and welcome, variations to the typical effective efforts to customize to strong patient preferences. That's the heart and soul of responsiveness.

Like any efficacious practice, preference accommodation boasts its contraindications, limitations, and boundaries. Rather than minimizing or hiding them, we opt to publicize them in an effort to match all clients to their optimal therapists and treatments. To do less is to compromise our ethical and professional responsibility to the best possible care.

9 TOWARD AN EVIDENCE-BASED BESPOKE PSYCHOTHERAPY

It is the client who knows what hurts, what directions to go, what problems are crucial, what experiences are deeply buried. It began to occur to me that unless I had a need to demonstrate my own cleverness and learning, I would do better to rely upon the client for the direction of movement in the process.
—Carl Rogers

If mental health professionals are to truly behave as scholar–professionals, then we will personalize psychotherapy to the singular patient in ways that accord with the compelling clinical experience (Chapter 3) and the cumulative research evidence (Chapter 2). That will generate evidence-based practices; in fact, that will lead to *best practices* in mental health. This is not our personal opinion nor gut intuition nor clinical lore; it is established fact.

In that future, we fully expect improvements in the research evidence, the Cooper–Norcross Inventory of Preferences (C-NIP), and the clinical methods of personalization. This chapter articulates and anticipates those future directions. The best is yet to come.

https://doi.org/10.1037/0000221-009
Personalizing Psychotherapy: Assessing and Accommodating Patient Preferences, by J. C. Norcross and M. Cooper

Although we endeavor to predict what will happen, as opposed to what we would like to happen, it is also possible to act in ways that can create a desirable future. Writing a book can turbocharge a particular movement forward, plan for the future, or even alter that future by forecasting its events. As stated in Chapter 1, George Orwell (1946/2005) wrote that the universal motivations of all writers were "to share an experience in which one feels is valuable and ought not to be missed" and "to push the world in a certain direction." For us, that direction is having all health professionals habitually assessing and accommodating patient preferences.

FUTURE OF PREFERENCE RESEARCH

Preference research in mental health has blossomed in recent years. Hundreds of studies have now been published, and their experimental or quasi-experimental designs permit causal conclusions. They show evidence of direct causal impact: Accommodating preferences results in reduced dropouts, enhanced alliances, and improved outcomes.

At the same time, as in any research enterprise, we can do better. Here are our top 10 ways to expand the research yield from preference research.

First, the recent meta-analyses only encompass English-language studies, with the preponderance of evidence coming from Western developed countries (Swift et al., 2019). The field needs more controlled studies from around the globe.

Second, the repeated finding of between-study heterogeneity in the preferences–outcomes link in the meta-analyses demonstrates a need for more fine-grained research. In particular, research is needed that measures the strength of specific preferences and/or examines the possibility that preference strength may vary according to the phase of treatment (Swift et al., 2018).

Third, although new measures of preference have appeared in the literature, psychometric study of those measures has been limited, and the extent to which they will be used clinically or in research is not yet known (Swift et al., 2019).

Fourth, practically all of the research to date has been conducted on individual patients and individual therapy. Studies on other therapy formats/ modalities are sorely required.

Fifth, closely related to the previous point, there is virtually no research to date on preferences, and their relation to outcomes, in work with children and young people. As the first step towards this end, measures are necessary that assess, in age-specific and developmentally sensitive ways, the treatment preferences of this client group.

Sixth, forthcoming research in psychotherapy preferences will progress from matching on macro-level preferences—such as medication versus psychotherapy or group versus individual treatment—to micro-level activity preferences—such as those identified in the C-NIP (Cooper, Norcross, et al., 2019). To some extent, this has already occurred in the research demonstrating the effectiveness of adapting psychotherapy to the client's ethnic background (Soto et al., 2018) and religious orientation (Hook et al., 2013). Those adaptations, like preference accommodation, work in general, but we do not know which particular therapist activities are the most effective. That, of course, is the typical trajectory of research: Start by investigating whether something works globally, then drill down to discern what works specifically.

Seventh, as with all psychotherapy research, future studies will intensify their focus on the specific effects of client diversity. A large body of research has sought to identify the preferences that racial and ethnic groups hold for psychotherapy (Swift et al., 2018). Much of this research has focused on clients' preferences for a therapist whose race and/or ethnicity matches their own. Meta-analytic reviews of this research have found a moderately strong effect size (ds in the 0.50 to 0.60 range) for such a match (Cabral & Smith, 2011; Soto et al., 2018). Other studies have indicated that racial and ethnic minority clients value other therapist characteristics (e.g., similar language and values) more strongly than demographic match (Bennett & BigFoot-Sipes, 1991; Soto et al., 2018; Stewart et al., 2013). For example, ethnic minority clients appear to value therapists' multicultural competence and use of cultural adaptations twice as strongly as they value racial or ethnic matching (Swift et al., 2015). Plus, little controlled research has examined preferences for psychotherapy based on client sexual orientation, socioeconomic status, or disability. These are all vital areas for future study.

Eighth, we require a clearer understanding of factors underlying client preferences. This includes establishing whether therapist directiveness and task focus, and past focus and insight orientation, are heterogeneous or homogenous dimensions (Cooper & Norcross, 2016). Research in this genre might benefit from drawing on theoretical models, as Berg and colleagues (2008) have done with coping styles. For instance, research into attachment styles (Ainsworth et al., 1978) could be utilized to develop and test the desire for warm support and other dimensions of interpersonal preferences. The interpersonal circumplex may prove a fruitful source for developing and refining preference measures (Horowitz et al., 2006).

Ninth, future research needs to explicate the mechanisms through which client preferences relate to clinical outcomes. In Chapter 3, we mapped out three potential pathways, but more inquiry will elucidate the relative weights of these processes and the circumstances under which some processes are more impactful than others. This also relates to our need to understand more about what preferences entail. For any individual, arriving at a preference requires a complex set of social, cognitive, and affective processes (Grund et al., 2018). A preference is far more complicated than just barking out what one desires.

That leads to our 10th and final key focus for research, and one that reflects the core theme of this book: Under which circumstances and with which patients will the assessment and accommodation of preferences be most (and least) valuable? Is it true, for instance, that clients with higher desires for control value preference assessment to a greater extent? Answering questions such as these will provide essential clinical guidance for tailoring the tailoring.

While most of these questions can only be answered through controlled quantitative research, in-depth qualitative studies will also prove essential in developing a deeper understanding of clients' experiences of preference assessment and accommodation (Trusty et al., 2019). How do clients feel about being asked about their preferences, and what are their reactions to having such preferences accommodated, or not accommodated? Likewise, recent attempts to investigate preference assessment using conversational analysis (e.g., Cantwell, 2017) suggest that this method may identify productive and unproductive means of eliciting preferences. For one example, *de-specifying*, in which the clinician scaffolds support for the client in making treatment decisions while minimizing deference effects, holds promise (Cantwell, 2017).

FUTURE OF THE C-NIP

We are more than a tad self-interested in the success of the C-NIP but can dispassionately summarize its research directions. Most immediately, we are completing several studies on the psychometric properties of the C-NIP. We have begun collecting additional data and reestablishing the provisional scale cutoff scores in light of the new results for representative laypersons and for in-therapy patients. The moderate internal consistency on some scales suggests that there may be a need for item refinement and scale development.

Further research is desirable to explore the clinical utility of the C-NIP. The research to date proves supportive (see Chapter 5), but more client and therapist ratings of its helpfulness is essential. Long-term studies linking the use of the C-NIP with improvement in patient outcomes should also be forthcoming.

The current measure is restricted to research and clinical use for individual counseling and psychotherapy in the United States and the United Kingdom, both Western, developed countries. Translations are available in a range of languages (www.c-nip.net/), but that will require restandardization and norming for individual countries.

The perpetual challenge is to balance the C-NIP's clinical utility with solid psychometrics. We desire a brief, multidimensional measure but one that boasts adequate reliability, validity, and normative samples.

FUTURE OF PERSONALIZATION

How can we ensure that health professionals regularly assess and accommodate their patients' preferences? And how can personalization of mental health services in general, and psychotherapy in particular, be enhanced in the coming decades? These critical questions of implementation and improvement occupy us here, in this final section of our final chapter.

Improving Implementation

Ensuring incorporation of patients' strong likes and dislikes in psychotherapy will require persistence and harmonization in training, practice, and policy.

Training

In terms of training, we will need to increasingly select students committed to human diversity and individual differences, educate them about the effectiveness of preference accommodation, train them to do so skillfully in graduate education, and then cultivate and maintain those competencies through clinical supervision (Chapter 7). That's a tall order in uncoordinated, even Byzantine, training curricula.

It will also prove vital to develop, for training purposes, a list of specific competencies in preference accommodation. Our current list in the training chapter (Chapter 7) is a provisional and personal effort; the profession as a whole will pinpoint which clinical behaviors are required and which are optional. And that will require research substantiation from qualitative and quantitative research.

Practice

Getting clinicians to use preference accommodation in daily practice, as explained in Chapter 7, consists of three distinct but overlapping steps: *dissemination* (raising awareness of available resources), *teaching* (the requisite core skills to competence), and *implementation* itself.

Research reviews have uniformly concluded that passive dissemination by itself exerts no significant effect on practitioner behavior (e.g., Fixsen et al., 2005; NHS Centre for Reviews and Dissemination, 1999). Passive dissemination of any evidence-based practice is not an evidence-based practice! Only the naive will believe that when research information becomes available, busy clinicians will access and then routinely apply it. Dissemination of information alone does not result in positive implementation outcomes (changes in practitioner behavior) or treatment outcomes (benefits to consumers). Thus, we should concentrate in the future on actively teaching the skills of preference accommodation (as covered in Chapter 7) and then on systems implementation—to which we now turn.

Training practitioners effectively leads to initial acquisition of skills but does not guarantee incorporation into daily practice. Nor does training individual practitioners automatically yield preference implementation throughout a unit or system of health care. But longer term, multilevel implementation can maximize practitioners' behavior change and thus enhance health care outcomes (Norcross et al., 2017).

That's the goal of *implementation science*: putting into routine practice an activity or program. It is an interdisciplinary field that investigates the methods that influence the integration of evidence-based interventions into practice settings and health care policy. Properly examining both individual behavior of practitioners and organizational systems of care, implementation scientists aim to reduce haphazard uptake of proven practices.

Here's what the research evidence—now totaling hundreds of individual studies—indicates will facilitate longer term, multilevel implementation (e.g., Fixsen et al., 2013; Greenhalgh et al., 2004; Mazzucchelli & Sanders, 2010; National Implementation Research Network, 2005; Norcross et al., 2017):

♦ Begin by conducting a readiness analysis of the system to identify factors likely to influence the proposed change (in this instance, preference assessment and accommodation).

♦ Secure the participation of local stakeholders and opinion leaders in the system or surrounding community.

♦ Collaborate with all key stakeholders, including clinicians, consumers, supervisors, insurance organizations, and mental health authorities (a process known as *co-creation*; Metz, 2015).

♦ Avoid single-bullet and time-limited trainings.

♦ Offer training to the entire staff.

♦ Provide training for trainers (and staff leaders) to maximize learning.

♦ Create peer support to build a culture of acceptance and support.

♦ Encourage the collection of clinical outcome data.

♦ Provide administrative and financial resources to sustain the changes.

♦ Use patient-specific reminders at the point of care for prompting the practice.

♦ Assess and track clinician fidelity.

♦ Monitor and evaluate the implementation.

♦ Insist that the new practices are conducted with fidelity before adapting to fit local needs; "first do it right, then do it differently."

♦ Provide follow-up training and supervision to reduce practitioner drift.

We will continue to offer workshops and website resources on personalizing psychotherapy to individual clinicians, to be sure, but we seek larger scale implementation to entire systems of care. There's a science to implementation and sustainability.

Think of systems implementation as a process of behavior change, akin to a patient moving through the stages of change: precontemplation, contemplation, preparation, action, and maintenance (Prochaska et al., 1992). Each stage represents a period of time, as well as a set of tasks needed for movement to the next stage. We will increasingly consider the organization's readiness to change because each stage and each system will require something a little different (Norcross et al., 2017).

Thus, like EBP itself, implementation science sensitively integrates the best research evidence, clinical expertise, and staff characteristics and preferences into deciding what works in each unique health care system. That is our goal in implementing wide-scale, system-wide adoption of preference accommodation. That will produce, as reviewed in Chapter 2, more effective behavioral health services for our patients and enhanced public health for the populace.

Policy

In terms of policy, professional organizations will need to incorporate the value of patient preferences and shared decision making into their ethical codes, practice guidelines, and EBP statements. This is certainly the case now in all of the major behavioral health professions in the United States and the United Kingdom.

Yet, we detect threats to the primacy of patient contributions in policy documents. EBP is universally defined by the three evidentiary sources of best available research, clinical expertise, and patient values and preferences. However, EBP is frequently misidentified or conflated in the literature with only the single pillar of research evidence. Patient input is marginalized, if not altogether neglected. By definition, the wholesale imposition of research without attending to the clinician or patient is not EBP; practitioners must insist on the proper use of the term and not let others commandeer the conversation.

Similarly, in promulgating treatment guidelines and compilations of best practices, practitioners must insist on the inclusion of client choice in determining what works best. "Nothing about us without us," as consumer groups advocate. It is a barely perceptible but slippery paternalistic slope when professionals begin to determine what is best for patients without shared decision making.

Improving Personalization

Improving personalization of psychotherapy can begin by consensually deciding on a single term for the process. The blizzard of terms (discussed in Chapter 1) begets confusion and diffusion; it confounds and obscures. Our favored term is *personalizing*, but we appreciate that others prefer *adaptations*, *individualization*, *responsiveness*, and a dozen others. But we need a common language, an Esperanto, or lingua franca to organize practice. The Rumpelstiltskin effect of naming something, and naming it consensually, grants us more power over it.

Clinical work and common sense also suggest that practitioners should increasingly focus on assessing and accommodating clients' *strong* likes and dislikes. Way too many research studies and clinical trainings attend to treatment preferences that may not exercise sufficient strength or valance to the patient. When researchers examine the effects of accommodating preferences for a single dimension, say, cognitive behavior therapy (CBT) or psychodynamic therapy, most patients will not possess strong preferences but are included in the study anyway. Clinical time is too precious to waste on middling likes. Better results will ensue from identifying and incorporating strong preferences.

Speaking of which, we are convinced that honoring what clients strongly *dis*like may be as effective as honoring what they strongly like. More research is required here, with specialized scales or inventories asking clients what they dislike or want to avoid in therapy, rather than what they favor. We continue to match to patients' likes, of course, but suspect that more clinical attention to the other pole may produce greater treatment outcomes.

Psychological assessment has matured from a single, standard battery of tests to focal, individualized evaluations; in a similar way, all psychological services will gravitate to more precise or personalized care (Norcross et al., 2016). This movement toward *precision psychotherapy*, paralleling precision medicine, is evidenced in *stepped care* and *specialized treatment matching*, among others.

Not all patients require the same intensity of mental health treatment; some will be sufficiently helped by a self-help computer program, some will benefit from a brief psychoeducational group, and still others will require long-term individual treatment from a graduate-trained professional. Stepped care attempts to maximize the effectiveness and efficiency of resource allocation, based on the belief (and evidence) that many individuals can successfully use a relatively small amount of information and support to help themselves resolve psychological problems in themselves and their family members (Cornish, 2020).

Psychotherapy is a powerful method and relationship, but in the past, it has been frequently applied in an inefficient, one-size-fits-all manner—by assigning the next patient to the next available therapist. In the future, clients will be progressively matched to therapies that accommodate their individual preferences, disorders, personalities, cultures, neuropsychological patterns, and so forth. The net result will be a more precise or personalized treatment that best fits the singular patient.

An example of this is the Personalized Advantage Index by DeRubeis and colleagues (2014) for the treatment of unipolar depression. The researchers identified a number of factors that can predict whether patients were more likely to do better with CBT or antidepressant medication. For instance, a greater number of stressful life events and lower levels of comorbid personality disorders indicated superior outcomes in CBT. They then showed that, for approximately 60% of patients, the allocation to an optimal treatment, based on the use of those factors, would have led to clinically significant improvements over allocation to a nonoptimal treatment. And, indeed, for these patients, there was a moderate difference for those who received their optimal treatment compared with those who received their nonoptimal treatment. In other words, the use of algorithms to predict which clients will do best in which treatments can probably contribute to improvements in outcomes.

The assessment of preferences is likely to play a key part in precision psychotherapies. That will entail the development of more sophisticated, complex, and accurate means of assessing preferences. A set of researchers (Crits-Christoph et al., 2017), to take one example, tested a process of *attribute-based preference assessment* in which patients were presented with 18 attributes of pharmacological and psychotherapeutic treatments for depression, such as having homework assignments and medication side effects. Patients then rated how strongly each attribute would affect their willingness to receive a treatment. Three statistical methods translated these attribute preferences into overall treatment preferences, with some evidence that greater matching was associated with reduced switching between treatments.

In the future, we expect—and we encourage—a synthesis of patient preferences with other demonstrably effective transdiagnostic treatment adaptions. Cases in point are cultural adaptations (Soto et al., 2018) and spiritual/religious accommodations (Hook et al., 2013). These treatment adaptations probably interconnect—if only in spirit and intent—and prove symbiotic, but we do not possess sufficient research to appraise whether the double or additive adaptation enhances treatment outcomes (Norcross & Wampold, 2019). But we believe that it does.

In the interminable debate on which psychotherapy works best, the dispassionate and evidence-based answer is, "It depends." It depends in particular on the client, including diagnostic features, but more important, transdiagnostic characteristics, such as preferences. Indeed, in our professional lifetimes, that is the sea change we have witnessed in our beloved art and science of psychotherapy. The therapist's principal question is no longer "What is my preferred theoretical orientation?" but rather "What does this particular client seek and prefer?"

IN CLOSING

The research evidence amounts to little if it is not enacted in practice and taught in graduate programs. We implore our colleagues to progress beyond the well-intended slogans and implement what we know works in responsiveness and simultaneously to avoid what does not. There's an exciting future for preference research, the C-NIP, routine implementation of preferences into practice and training, as well as personalized or precision treatments.

When practitioners successfully do so, a bevy of benefits will almost certainly accrue. We deepen our commitment to ethical, evidence-based, and cultural diversity mandates. We transcend the limited and divisive "diagnosis only" approach to psychotherapy. We narrow the gap between research and practice. We embrace the clinical reality that patients respond differently. We rediscover the individual differences that distinguish our field. We reorient from internecine conflict to patient benefit. And, most consequential, we become demonstrably more effective with our clients. That's the compelling case for personalizing psychotherapy.

COOPER–NORCROSS INVENTORY OF PREFERENCES (C-NIP)

Cooper–Norcross Inventory of Preferences (C-NIP) v1.1

On each of the items below, please indicate your preferences for how a psycho-therapist or counsellor should work with you by circling a number. A 3 indicates a *strong* preference in that direction, 2 indicates a *moderate* preference in that direction, 1 indicates a *slight* preference in that direction, 0 indicates no preference in either direction/an equally strong preference in both directions.

'I would like the therapist to...'

1. Focus on specific goals		No or equal preference				Not focus on specific goals
3	2	1	0	-1	-2	-3

2. Give structure to the therapy		No or equal preference				Allow the therapy to be unstructured
3	2	1	0	-1	-2	-3

3. Teach me skills to deal with my problems		No or equal preference				Not teach me skills to deal with my problems
3	2	1	0	-1	-2	-3

4. Give me 'homework' to do		No or equal preference				Not give me 'homework' to do
3	2	1	0	-1	-2	-3

5. Take a lead in therapy		No or equal preference				Allow me to take a lead in therapy
3	2	1	0	-1	-2	-3

Scale 1. If score is 8 to 15 then strong preference for therapist directiveness. If score is -2 to 7 then no strong preference. If score is -3 to -15 then strong preference for client directiveness.

(continues)

6. Encourage me to go into difficult emotions		No or equal preference			Not encourage me to go into difficult emotions	
3	2	1	0	-1	-2	-3

7. Talk with me about the therapy relationship		No or equal preference			Not talk with me about the therapy relationship	
3	2	1	0	-1	-2	-3

8. Focus on the relationship between us		No or equal preference			Not focus on the relationship between us	
3	2	1	0	-1	-2	-3

9. Encourage me to express strong feelings		No or equal preference			Not encourage me to express strong feelings	
3	2	1	0	-1	-2	-3

10. Focus mainly on my feelings		No or equal preference			Focus mainly on my thoughts	
3	2	1	0	-1	-2	-3

Scale 2. If score is 7 to 15 then strong preference for emotional intensity. If score is 0 to 6 then no strong preference. If score is -15 to -1 then strong preference for emotional reserve.

11. Focus on my life in the past		No or equal preference			Focus on my life in the present	
3	2	1	0	-1	-2	-3

12. Help me reflect on my childhood		No or equal preference			Help me reflect on my adulthood	
3	2	1	0	-1	-2	-3

13. Focus on my past		No or equal preference			Focus on my future	
3	2	1	0	-1	-2	-3

Scale 3. If score is 3 to 9 then strong preference for past orientation. If score is -2 to 2 then no strong preference. If score is -3 to -9 then strong preference for present orientation.

14. Be gentle		No or equal preference			Be challenging	
3	2	1	0	-1	-2	-3

15. Be supportive		No or equal preference			Be confrontational	
3	2	1	0	-1	-2	-3

16. Not interrupt me		No or equal preference			Interrupt me and keep me focused	
3	2	1	0	-1	-2	-3

17. Not be challenging of my own beliefs and views		No or equal preference			Be challenging of my own beliefs and views	
3	2	1	0	-1	-2	-3

18. Support my behaviour unconditionally		No or equal preference			Challenge my behaviour if they think it's wrong	
3	2	1	0	-1	-2	-3

Scale 4. If score is 4 to 15 then strong preference for warm support. If score is -3 to 3 then no strong preference. If score is -4 to -15 then strong preference for focused challenge.

Additional client preferences for exploration and consideration (as appropriate to service provision)

Do you have a *strong* preference for:

- A therapist of a particular **gender, race/ethnicity, sexual orientation, religion,** or **other personal characteristic**?

- A therapist/counsellor who speaks a **specific language** that is most comfortable for you?

- **Modality** of therapy: such as individual, couple, family, or group therapy?

- **Orientation** of therapy: such as psychodynamic, cognitive, person-centered, or other?

- **Number** of therapy sessions: such as four, dependent on review, open-minded, or other?

- **Length** of therapy sessions: such as 50 mins, 60 mins, 90 mins or other?

- **Frequency** of therapy: such as twice weekly, weekly, monthly, ad hoc or other?

- **Medication,** psychotherapy, or both in combination?

- Use of **self-help** books, self-help groups, or computer programs in addition to therapy?

- **Any other** strong preferences that come to mind? (and do raise them at any point in therapy)

- What would you most **dislike** or **despise** happening in your therapy or counselling?

Note. Licensed under CC BY-ND 4.0. Reprinted with permission.

References

Ainsworth, M. D. S., Blehar, M. C., Waters, E., & Wall, S. (1978). *Patterns of attachment: A psychological study of the strange situation*. Erlbaum.

Allen, G. J., Szollos, S. J., & Williams, B. E. (1986). Doctoral students' comparative evaluations of best and worst psychotherapy supervision. *Professional Psychology: Research and Practice*, *17*(2), 91–99. https://doi.org/10.1037/0735-7028.17.2.91

American Psychiatric Association. (2006). *American Psychiatric Association practice guidelines for the treatment of psychiatric disorder compendium*. American Psychiatric Publishing.

American Psychological Association. (2017). *Ethical principles of psychologists and code of conduct* (2002, amended effective June 1, 2010 and January 1, 2017). https://www.apa.org/ethics/code/index.aspx

American Psychological Association, Presidential Task Force on Evidence-Based Practice. (2006). Evidence-based practice in psychology. *American Psychologist*, *61*(4), 271–285. https://doi.org/10.1037/0003-066X.61.4.271

Andrew, K. (2011). *Client narratives of perceived helpful factors of person centered therapy* [Unpublished doctoral dissertation]. University of Strathclyde/Glasgow Caledonian University.

Auerbach, A. H., & Johnson, M. (1977). Research on the therapist's level of experience. In A. S. Gurman & A. M. Razin (Eds.), *Effective psychotherapy: A handbook of research* (pp. 84–102). Pergamon.

Aylindar, S. (2014). *The Therapy Personalisation Form* [Unpublished doctoral dissertation]. University of Strathclyde/Glasgow Caledonian University.

Barkham, M., Hardy, G. E., & Mellor-Clark, J. (Eds.). (2010). *Developing and delivering practice-based evidence: A guide for the psychological therapies*. Wiley. https://doi.org/10.1002/9780470687994

Barlow, D. H. (Ed.). (2014). *Clinical handbook of psychological disorders: A step-by-step treatment manual* (5th ed.). Guilford Press. https://doi.org/10.1093/oxfordhb/9780199328710.001.0001

Becker, S. J., Helseth, S. A., Frank, H. E., Escobar, K., & Weeks, B. (2018). Parent preferences and experiences with psychological treatment: Results from a direct-to-consumer survey using the marketing mix framework. *Professional Psychology: Research and Practice, 49*(2), 167–176. https://doi.org/10.1037/pro0000186

Bedi, N., Chilvers, C., Churchill, R., Dewey, M., Duggan, C., Fielding, K., Gretton, V., Miller, P., Harrison, G., Lee, A., & Williams, I. (2000). Assessing effectiveness of treatment of depression in primary care: Partially randomised preference trial. *The British Journal of Psychiatry, 177*(4), 312–318. https://doi.org/10.1192/bjp.177.4.312

Benbassat, J., Pilpel, D., & Tidhar, M. (1998). Patients' preferences for participation in clinical decision making: A review of published surveys. *Behavioral Medicine, 24*(2), 81–88. https://doi.org/10.1080/08964289809596384

Bennett, S. K., & BigFoot-Sipes, D. S. (1991). American Indian and White college student preferences for counselor characteristics. *Journal of Counseling Psychology, 38*(4), 440–445. https://doi.org/10.1037/0022-0167.38.4.440

Berg, A. L., Sandahl, C., & Clinton, D. (2008). The relationship of treatment preferences and experiences to outcome in generalized anxiety disorder (GAD). *Psychology and Psychotherapy: Theory, Research and Practice, 81*(3), 247–259. https://doi.org/10.1348/147608308X297113

Berlin, I. (1958). Two concepts of liberty. In H. Hardy (Ed.), *Liberty* (pp. 166–217). Oxford University Press.

Bernal, G. E., & Domenech Rodríguez, M. M. (Eds.). (2012). *Cultural adaptations: Tools for evidence-based practice with diverse populations*. American Psychological Association. https://doi.org/10.1037/13752-000

Beutler, L. E. (2011). Prescriptive matching and systematic treatment selection. In J. C. Norcross, G. R. VandenBos, & D. K. Freedheim (Eds.), *History of psychotherapy: Continuity and change* (2nd ed., pp. 402–407). American Psychological Association. https://doi.org/10.1037/12353-019

Beutler, L. E., & Clarkin, J. (1990). *Systematic treatment selection: Toward targeted therapeutic interventions*. Brunner/Mazel.

Beutler, L. E., Machado, P. P. P., & Neufeldt, S. A. (1994). Therapist variables. In A. E. Bergin & S. L. Garfield (Eds.), *Handbook of psychotherapy and behavior change* (4th ed., pp. 229–269). Wiley.

Beutler, L. E., Mahoney, M. J., Norcross, J. C., Prochaska, J. O., Sollod, R. M., & Robertson, M. (1987). Training integrative/eclectic psychotherapists II. *International Journal of Eclectic Psychotherapy, 6*(3), 296–332.

Bion, W. R. (1967). Notes on memory and desire. *Psychoanalytic Forum, 2*, 279–281.

Blatt, S. J., & Felsen, I. (1993). Different kinds of folks may need different kinds of strokes: The effect of patients' characteristics on therapeutic process and outcome. *Psychotherapy Research, 3*(4), 245–259. https://doi.org/10.1080/10503309312331333829

Bohart, A. C. (2005). Evidence-based psychotherapy means evidence-informed, not evidence-driven. *Journal of Contemporary Psychotherapy, 35*(1), 39–53. https://doi.org/10.1007/s10879-005-0802-8

Bohart, A., & Tallman, K. (1999). *How clients make therapy work: The process of active self-healing.* American Psychological Association. https://doi.org/10.1037/10323-000

Bohart, A. C., & Wade, A. G. (2013). The client in psychotherapy. In M. J. Lambert (Ed.), *Bergin and Garfield's handbook of psychotherapy and behavior change* (6th ed., pp. 219–257). Wiley.

Bordin, E. S. (1979). The generalizability of the psychoanalytic concept of the working alliance. *Psychotherapy: Theory, Research & Practice, 16*(3), 252–260. https://doi.org/10.1037/h0085885

Borrell-Carrió, F., Suchman, A. L., & Epstein, R. M. (2004). The biopsychosocial model 25 years later: Principles, practice, and scientific inquiry. *Annals of Family Medicine, 2*(6), 576–582. https://doi.org/10.1370/afm.245

Boswell, J. F., Constantino, M. J., Oswald, J. M., Bugatti, M., Goodwin, B., & Yucel, R. (2018). Mental health care consumers' relative valuing of clinician performance information. *Journal of Consulting and Clinical Psychology, 86*(4), 301–308. https://doi.org/10.1037/ccp0000264

Bowens, M., & Cooper, M. (2012). Development of a client feedback tool: A qualitative study of therapists' experiences of using the Therapy Personalisation Forms. *European Journal of Psychotherapy and Counselling, 14*(1), 47–62. https://doi.org/10.1080/13642537.2012.652392

Bragesjö, M., Clinton, D., & Sandell, R. (2004). The credibility of psychodynamic, cognitive and cognitive-behavioural psychotherapy in a randomly selected sample of the general public. *Psychology and Psychotherapy: Theory, Research and Practice, 77*(3), 297–307. https://doi.org/10.1348/1476083041839358

British Association for Counselling and Psychotherapy. (2018). *Ethical framework for the counselling professions.* https://www.abdn.ac.uk/students/documents/bacp-ethical-framework-for-the-counselling-professions-2018.pdf

Bucky, S. T., Marques, S., Daly, J., Alley, J., & Karp, A. (2010). Supervision characteristics related to the supervisory working alliance as rated by doctoral-level supervisees. *The Clinical Supervisor, 29*(2), 149–163. https://doi.org/10.1080/07325223.2010.519270

Burger, J. M., & Cooper, H. M. (1979). The desirability of control. *Motivation and Emotion, 3*(4), 381–393. https://doi.org/10.1007/BF00994052

Cabral, R. R., & Smith, T. B. (2011). Racial/ethnic matching of clients and therapists in mental health services: A meta-analytic review of preferences, perceptions, and outcomes. *Journal of Counseling Psychology, 58*(4), 537–554. https://doi.org/10.1037/a0025266

Cantwell, S. (2017). *Talk about what might be helpful: Relating meta-therapeutic dialogue to concrete interactions and exploring the relevance for therapeutic practice* [Unpublished doctoral dissertation]. University of Roehampton.

Caplandies, F. C., Brown, J. A., Murray, A. B., Rose, J. P., & Geers, A. L. (2018). Choice and perceptions of exercise: A test of three moderating variables. *Psychology of Sport and Exercise, 38,* 47–55. https://doi.org/10.1016/j.psychsport.2018.05.012

Captari, L. E., Hook, J. N., Hoyt, W., Davis, D. E., McElroy-Heltzel, S. E., & Worthington, E. L., Jr. (2018). Integrating clients' religion and spirituality within psychotherapy: A comprehensive meta-analysis. *Journal of Clinical Psychology, 74*(11), 1938–1951. https://doi.org/10.1002/jclp.22681

Castonguay, L., & Hill, C. E. (Eds.). (2017). *How and why are some therapists better than others? Understanding therapist effects.* American Psychological Association. https://doi.org/10.1037/0000034-000

Charles, C. A., Whelan, T., Gafni, A., Willan, A., & Farrell, S. (2003). Shared treatment decision making: What does it mean to physicians? *Journal of Clinical Oncology, 21*(5), 932–936. https://doi.org/10.1200/JCO.2003.05.057

Chickering, A. W., & Gamson, Z. F. (1987, March). Seven principles for good practice in undergraduate education. *AAHE Bulletin, 1987,* 3–7. https://files.eric.ed.gov/fulltext/ED282491.pdf

Chu, B. C., & Kendall, P. C. (2009). Therapist responsiveness to child engagement: Flexibility within manual-based CBT for anxious youth. *Journal of Clinical Psychology, 65*(7), 736–754. https://doi.org/10.1002/jclp.20582

Chu, J., & Leino, A. (2017). Advancement in the maturing science of cultural adaptations of evidence-based interventions. *Journal of Consulting and Clinical Psychology, 85*(1), 45–57. https://doi.org/10.1037/ccp0000145

Clarkin, J. F., & Levy, K. N. (2004). The influence of client variables on psychotherapy. In M. J. Lambert (Ed.), *Handbook of psychotherapy and behavior change* (5th ed., pp. 194–226). Wiley.

Cochrane, A. L. (1979). 1931–1971: A critical review with particular reference to the medical profession. In G. Teeling-Smith (Ed.), *Medicines for the year 2000* (pp. 1–11). Office of Health Economics.

Cohen, J. (1988). *Statistical power analysis for the behavioral sciences* (2nd ed.). Erlbaum.

Cooper, M. (2008). *Essential research findings in counselling and psychotherapy: The facts are friendly.* SAGE.

Cooper, M. (2009). Welcoming the Other: Actualising the humanistic ethic at the core of counselling psychology practice. *Counselling Psychology Review, 24*(3&4), 119–129.

Cooper, M. (2015). *Existential psychotherapy and counselling: Contributions to a pluralistic practice.* SAGE.

Cooper, M. (2017). *Existential therapies* (2nd ed.). SAGE.

Cooper, M., Di Malta, G. S., & Oza, M. (2020). *CREST Clinic data* [Unpublished raw data].

Cooper, M., & McLeod, J. (2007). A pluralistic framework for counselling and psychotherapy: Implications for research. *Counselling & Psychotherapy Research, 7*(3), 135–143. https://doi.org/10.1080/14733140701566282

Cooper, M., & McLeod, J. (2011). *Pluralistic counselling and psychotherapy.* SAGE.

Cooper, M., Messow, C., McConnachie, A., Freire, E., Elliott, R., Heard, D., Williams, C., & Morrison, J. (2018). Patient preference as a predictor of outcomes in a pilot trial of person-centered counselling versus low-intensity cognitive behavioural therapy for persistent sub-threshold and mild depression. *Counselling Psychology Quarterly, 31*(4), 460–476. https://doi.org/10.1080/09515070.2017.1329708

Cooper, M., & Norcross, J. C. (2016). A brief, multidimensional measure of clients' therapy preferences: The Cooper–Norcross Inventory of Preferences (C-NIP). *International Journal of Clinical and Health Psychology, 16*(1), 87–98. https://doi.org/10.1016/j.ijchp.2015.08.003

Cooper, M., Norcross, J. C., Raymond-Barker, B., & Hogan, T. P. (2017). [Unpublished raw data on the Cooper–Norcross Inventory of Preferences]. University of Roehampton.

Cooper, M., Norcross, J. C., Raymond-Barker, B., & Hogan, T. P. (2019). Psychotherapy preferences of laypersons and mental health professionals: Whose therapy is it? *Psychotherapy, 56*(2), 205–216. https://doi.org/10.1037/pst0000226

Cooper, M., O'Hara, M., Schmid, P. F., & Bohart, A. C. (Eds.). (2013). *The handbook of person-centred psychotherapy and counselling* (2nd ed.). Palgrave.

Cooper, M., van Rijn, B., Chryssafidou, E., & Stiles, W. B. (2020). *Activity preferences in psychotherapy: What do patients want and how does this relate to outcomes?* [Manuscript in preparation]. Department of Psychology, University of Roehampton.

Cooper, M., Watson, J. C., & Hölldampf, D. (Eds.). (2010). *Person-centred and experiential therapies work: A review of the research on counseling, psychotherapy and related practices.* PCCS Books.

Cooper, M., Wild, C., van Rijn, B., Ward, T., McLeod, J., Cassar, S., Antoniou, P., Michael, C., Michalitsi, M., & Sreenath, S. (2015). Pluralistic therapy for depression: Acceptability, outcomes and helpful aspects in a multisite open-label trail. *Counselling Psychology Review, 30*(1), 6–20.

Cornish, P. (2020). *Stepped care 2.0: A paradigm shift in mental health.* Springer.

Coulter, A., & Collins, A. (2011). *Making shared decision-making a reality: No decision about me, without me.* The King's Fund.

Coursol, A., & Sipps, G. J. (1986). Examination of the unintentional effect of stimulus medium and context on preference for psychotherapy. *Journal of Clinical Psychology, 42*(2), 280–286. https://doi.org/10.1002/1097-4679(198603)42:2%3C280::AID-JCLP2270420209%3E3.0.CO;2-I

Crits-Christoph, P., Gallop, R., Diehl, C. K., Yin, S., & Gibbons, M. B. C. (2017). Methods for incorporating patient preferences for treatments of depression in community mental health settings. *Administration and Policy in Mental Health and Mental Health Services Research, 44*(5), 735–746. https://doi.org/10.1007/s10488-016-0746-1

Cucciare, M. A., Weingardt, K. R., & Villafranca, S. (2008). Using blended learning to implement evidence-based psychotherapies. *Clinical Psychology: Science and Practice, 15*(4), 299–307. https://doi.org/10.1111/j.1468-2850.2008.00141.x

Cucherat, M., Haugh, M. C., Gooch, M., Boissel, J.-P., & the Homeopathic Medicines Research Advisory Group. (2000). Evidence of clinical efficacy of homeopathy: A meta-analysis of clinical trials. *European Journal of Clinical Pharmacology, 56*(1), 27–33. https://doi.org/10.1007/s002280050716

DeRubeis, R. J., Cohen, Z. D., Forand, N. R., Fournier, J. C., Gelfand, L. A., & Lorenzo-Luaces, L. (2014). The Personalized Advantage Index: Translating research on prediction into individualized treatment recommendations. A demonstration. *PLoS ONE, 9*(1), e83875. https://doi.org/10.1371/journal.pone.0083875

Devine, D. A., & Fernald, P. S. (1973). Outcome effects of receiving a preferred, randomly assigned, or nonpreferred therapy. *Journal of Consulting and Clinical Psychology, 41*(1), 104–107. https://doi.org/10.1037/h0035617

Dimeff, L. A., Koerner, K., Woodcock, E. A., Beadnell, B., Brown, M. Z., Skutch, J. M., Paves, A. P., Bazinet, A., & Harned, M. S. (2009). Which training method works best? A randomized controlled trial comparing three methods of training clinicians in dialectical behavior therapy skills. *Behaviour Research and Therapy, 47*(11), 921–930. https://doi.org/10.1016/j.brat.2009.07.011

Dockett, L. (2018). The case of giving your client the reins: Does the therapist really know best? *Psychotherapy Networker.* https://www.psychotherapynetworker.org/blog/details/1383/the-case-for-giving-your-client-the-reins

Duckro, P. N., & George, C. E. (1979). Effects of failure to meet client preference in a counseling interview analogue. *Journal of Counseling Psychology, 26*(1), 9–14. https://doi.org/10.1037/0022-0167.26.1.9

Dugas, M., Shorten, A., Dubé, E., Wassef, M., Bujold, E., & Chaillet, N. (2012). Decision aid tools to support women's decision making in pregnancy and birth: A systematic review and meta-analysis. *Social Science & Medicine, 74*(12), 1968–1978. https://doi.org/10.1016/j.socscimed.2012.01.041

Duncan, B. L., & Miller, S. D. (2008). *The Outcome and Session Rating Scales: The revised administration and scoring manual, including the Child Outcome Rating Scale.* Institute for the Study of Therapeutic Change.

Duncan, B. L., Miller, S. D., Wampold, B. E., & Hubble, M. A. (Eds.). (2010). *The heart and soul of change in psychotherapy: Delivering what works in therapy* (2nd ed.). American Psychological Association.

Duncan, E., Best, C., & Hagen, S. (2010). Shared decision making interventions for people with mental health conditions. *Cochrane Database of Systematic Reviews, 2010*(1), CD007297. https://doi.org/10.1002/14651858.CD007297.pub2

Durand, M.-A., Carpenter, L., Dolan, H., Bravo, P., Mann, M., Bunn, F., & Elwyn, G. (2014). Do interventions designed to support shared decision-making reduce health inequalities? A systematic review and meta-analysis. *PLoS ONE, 9*(4), e94670. https://doi.org/10.1371/journal.pone.0094670

Edwards, C. J., Beutler, L. E., & Someah, K. (2019). Reactance level. In J. C. Norcross & B. E. Wampold (Eds.), *Psychotherapy relationships that work: Vol. 2. Evidence-based therapist responsiveness* (3rd ed., pp. 188–211). Oxford University Press. https://doi.org/10.1093/med-psych/9780190843960.003.0007

Elkin, I., Yamaguchi, J. L., Arnkoff, D. B., Glass, C. R., Sotsky, S. M., & Krupnick, J. L. (1999). "Patient–treatment fit" and early engagement in therapy. *Psychotherapy Research*, *9*(4), 437–451. https://doi.org/10.1080/10503309912331332851

Elliott, R. (2000). *The Session Effectiveness Scale* [Unpublished questionnaire]. Department of Psychology, University of Toledo.

Eubanks, C. F., Muran, J. C., & Safran, J. D. (2018). Alliance rupture repair: A meta-analysis. *Psychotherapy*, *55*(4), 508–519. https://doi.org/10.1037/pst0000185

Farber, B. A., & Doolin, E. M. (2011). Positive regard. *Psychotherapy*, *48*(1), 58–64. https://doi.org/10.1037/a0022141

Festinger, L. (1957). *A theory of cognitive dissonance* (Vol. 2). Stanford University Press.

Fischer, C. T. (1970). The testee as co-evaluator. *Journal of Counseling Psychology*, *17*(1), 70–76. https://doi.org/10.1037/h0028630

Fixsen, D., Blasé, K., Metz, A., & Van Dyke, M. (2013). Statewide implementation of evidence-based programs. *Exceptional Children*, *79*(3), 213–230. https://doi.org/10.1177/001440291307900206

Fixsen, D., Naoom, S., Blase, K., Friedman, R., & Wallace, F. (2005). *Implementation research: A synthesis of the literature*. National Implementation Research Network.

Flückiger, C., Del Re, A. C., Wampold, B. E., & Horvath, A. O. (2018). The alliance in adult psychotherapy: A meta-analytic synthesis. *Psychotherapy*, *55*(4), 316–340. https://doi.org/10.1037/pst0000172

Fox, J., Close, S. R., Rose, J. P., & Geers, A. L. (2016). Identifying when choice helps: Clarifying the relationships between choice making, self-construal, and pain. *Journal of Behavioral Medicine*, *39*(3), 527–536. https://doi.org/10.1007/s10865-015-9708-4

Frances, A., Clarkin, J., & Perry, S. (1984). *Differential therapeutics in psychiatry*. Brunner/Mazel.

Freire, E., Williams, C., Messow, C.-M., Cooper, M., Elliott, R., McConnachie, A., Walker, A., Heard, D., & Morrison, J. (2015). Counselling versus low-intensity cognitive behavioural therapy for persistent sub-threshold and mild depression (CLICD): A pilot/feasibility randomised controlled trial. *BMC Psychiatry*, *15*(1), 197. https://doi.org/10.1186/s12888-015-0582-y

Freire, P. (2018). *Pedagogy of the oppressed: 50th anniversary edition* (4th ed.). Bloomsbury Academic.

Friedlander, M. L. (2015). Use of relational strategies to repair alliance ruptures: How responsive supervisors train responsive psychotherapists. *Psychotherapy*, *52*(2), 174–179. https://doi.org/10.1037/a0037044

Friedrichs, A., Spies, M., Härter, M., & Buchholz, A. (2016). Patient preferences and shared decision making in the treatment of substance use disorders:

A systematic review of the literature. *PLoS ONE, 11*(1), e0145817. https://doi.org/10.1371/journal.pone.0145817

Frövenholt, J., Bragesjö, M., Clinton, D., & Sandell, R. (2007). How do experiences of psychiatric care affect the perceived credibility of different forms of psychotherapy? *Psychology and Psychotherapy: Theory, Research and Practice, 80*(2), 205–215. https://doi.org/10.1348/147608306X116098

Geers, A. L., Rose, J. P., Fowler, S. L., Rasinski, H. M., Brown, J. A., & Helfer, S. G. (2013). Why does choice enhance treatment effectiveness? Using placebo treatments to demonstrate the role of personal control. *Journal of Personality and Social Psychology, 105*(4), 549–566. https://doi.org/10.1037/a0034005

Geller, J. D., Norcross, J. C., & Orlinsky, D. E. (Eds.). (2005). *The psychotherapist's own psychotherapy: Patient and clinician perspectives.* Oxford University Press. https://doi.org/10.1093/med:psych/9780195133943.001.0001

Gibson, A., Cooper, M., Rae, J., & Hayes, J. (2020). Clients' experiences of shared decision making in an integrative psychotherapy for depression. *Journal of Evaluation in Clinical Practice, 26*(2), 559–568. https://doi.org/10.1111/jep.13320

Gnambs, T., & Kaspar, K. (2015). Disclosure of sensitive behaviors across self-administered survey modes: A meta-analysis. *Behavior Research Methods, 47*(4), 1237–1259. https://doi.org/10.3758/s13428-014-0533-4

Goates-Jones, M., & Hill, C. E. (2008). Treatment preference, treatment-preference match, and psychotherapist credibility: Influence on session outcome and preference shift. *Psychotherapy, 45*(1), 61–74. https://doi.org/10.1037/0033-3204.45.1.61

Greenberg, R. P. (2016). The rebirth of psychosocial importance in a drug-filled world. *American Psychologist, 71*(8), 781–791. https://doi.org/10.1037/amp0000054

Greenhalgh, T., Robert, G., Macfarlane, F., Bate, P., & Kyriakidou, O. (2004). Diffusion of innovations in service organizations: Systematic review and recommendations. *Milbank Quarterly, 82*(4), 581–629. https://doi.org/10.1111/j.0887-378X.2004.00325.x

Grund, A., Fries, S., & Rheinberg, F. (2018). Know your preferences: Self-regulation as need-congruent goal selection. *Review of General Psychology, 22*(4), 437–451. https://doi.org/10.1037/gpr0000159

Gurman, A. S. (1973). Effects of therapist and patient mood on the therapeutic functioning of high- and low-facilitative therapists. *Journal of Consulting and Clinical Psychology, 40*(1), 48–58. https://doi.org/10.1037/h0034032

Guyatt, G., Rennie, D., Meade, M. O., & Cook, D. J. (2008). *Users' guides to the medical literature: Essentials of evidence-based clinical practice* (2nd ed.). McGraw-Hill.

Handelzalts, J. E., & Keinan, G. (2010). The effect of choice between test anxiety treatment options on treatment outcomes. *Psychotherapy Research, 20*(1), 100–112. https://doi.org/10.1080/10503300903121106

Hanson, W. E., Claiborn, C. D., & Kerr, B. (1997). Differential effects of two test-interpretation styles in counseling: A field study. *Journal of Counseling Psychology, 44*(4), 400–405. https://doi.org/10.1037/0022-0167.44.4.400

Hatcher, R. L. (2015). Interpersonal competencies: Responsiveness, technique, and training in psychotherapy. *American Psychologist, 70*(8), 747–757. https://doi.org/10.1037/a0039803

Hatchett, G. T. (2015a). Development of the Preferences for College Counseling Inventory. *Journal of College Counseling, 18*(1), 37–48. https://doi.org/10.1002/j.2161-1882.2015.00067.x

Hatchett, G. T. (2015b). *Preferences for College Counselling Measure development notes* [Unpublished manuscript]. Department of Counseling, Social Work, and Leadership, Northern Kentucky University.

Hayes, D., Town, R., Lemoniatis, E., Moore, A., & James, R. (2018). *i-THRIVE grids.* http://www.implementingthrive.org/i-thrive-grids/

The Health Foundation. (2012). *Helping people share decision making.* https://www.health.org.uk/publications/helping-people-share-decision-making

The Health Foundation. (2014). *Person-centered care: From ideas to action.* https://www.health.org.uk/publications/person-centred-care-from-ideas-to-action

Henry, W. E., Sims, J. H., & Spray, S. L. (1971). *The fifth profession: Becoming a psychotherapist.* Jossey-Bass.

Hill, C. E., Spiegel, S., Hoffman, M. A., Kivlighan, D., Jr., & Gelso, C. (2017). Therapist expertise in psychotherapy revisited. *The Counseling Psychologist, 45*(1), 7–53. https://doi.org/10.1177/0011000016641192

Hogan, R. A. (1964). Issues and approaches in supervision. *Psychotherapy: Theory, Research & Practice, 1*(3), 139–141. https://doi.org/10.1037/h0088589

Holloway, E. L., & Wampold, B. E. (1986). Relation between conceptual level and counseling-related tasks: A meta-analysis. *Journal of Counseling Psychology, 33*(3), 310–319. https://doi.org/10.1037/0022-0167.33.3.310

Hong, N., Cornacchio, D., Pettit, J. W., & Comer, J. S. (2019). Coal-mining canaries in clinical psychology: Getting better at identifying early signals of treatment nonresponse. *Clinical Psychological Science, 7*(6), 1207–1221. https://doi.org/10.1177/2167702619858111

Hook, J. N., Captari, L. E., Hoyt, W., Davis, D. E., McElroy, S. E., & Worthington, E. L. (2019). Religion and spirituality. In J. C. Norcross & B. E. Wampold (Eds.), *Psychotherapy relationships that work: Vol. 2. Evidence-based therapist responsiveness* (3rd ed., p. 212). Oxford University Press. https://doi.org/10.1093/med-psych/9780190843960.003.0008

Hook, J. N., Davis, D. E., Owen, J., Worthington, E. L., Jr., & Utsey, S. O. (2013). Cultural humility: Measuring openness to culturally diverse clients. *Journal of Counseling Psychology, 60*(3), 353–366. https://doi.org/10.1037/a0032595

Horowitz, L. M., Wilson, K. R., Turan, B., Zolotsev, P., Constantino, M. J., & Henderson, L. (2006). How interpersonal motives clarify the meaning of interpersonal behavior: A revised circumplex model. *Personality and Social Psychology Review, 10*(1), 67–86. https://doi.org/10.1207/s15327957pspr1001_4

Horvath, A. O. (1992). *Working Alliance Inventory*. http://wai.profhorvath.com/

Institute of Medicine. (2001). *Crossing the quality chasm: A new health system for the 21st century*. National Academy Press.

James, W. (1987). *William James: Writings 1902–1910*. Library of America. (Original work published 1909)

James, W. (1996). *A pluralistic universe*. University of Nebraska. (Original work published 1909)

Kayrouz, R., & Hansen, S. (2020). I don't believe in miracles: Using the ecological validity model to adapt the miracle question to match the client's cultural preferences and characteristics. *Professional Psychology: Research and Practice, 51*(3), 223–236. https://doi.org/10.1037/pro0000283

Kent, D., Paulus, J., Ahmed, M., & Whicher, D. (Eds.). (2019). *Caring for the individual patient: Understanding heterogeneous treatment effects*. National Academy of Medicine.

Kerns, R. D., Burns, J. W., Shulman, M., Jensen, M. P., Nielson, W. R., Czlapinski, R., Dallas, M. I., Chatkoff, D., Sellinger, J., Heapy, A., & Rosenberger, P. (2014). Can we improve cognitive-behavioral therapy for chronic back pain treatment engagement and adherence? A controlled trial of tailored versus standard therapy. *Health Psychology, 33*(9), 938–947. https://doi.org/10.1037/a0034406

King, M., Sibbald, B., Ward, E., Bower, P., Lloyd, M., Gabbay, M., & Byford, S. (2000). Randomised controlled trial of non-directive counselling, cognitive-behaviour therapy and usual general practitioner care in the management of depression as well as mixed anxiety and depression in primary care. *Health Technology Assessment, 4*(19), 1–83. https://doi.org/10.3310/hta4190

Knops, A. M., Legemate, D. A., Goossens, A., Bossuyt, P. M., & Ubbink, D. T. (2013). Decision aids for patients facing a surgical treatment decision: A systematic review and meta-analysis. *Annals of Surgery, 257*(5), 860–866. https://doi.org/10.1097/SLA.0b013e3182864fd6

Koocher, G. P., & Keith-Spiegel, P. (2016). *Ethics in psychology and the mental health professions: Standards and cases* (4th ed.). Oxford University Press.

Kramer, U., & Stiles, W. B. (2015). The responsiveness problem in psychotherapy: A review of proposed solutions. *Clinical Psychology: Science and Practice, 22*(3), 277–295. https://doi.org/10.1111/cpsp.12107

Krebs, P., Norcross, J. C., Nicholson, J. M., & Prochaska, J. O. (2018). Stages of change and psychotherapy outcomes: A review and meta-analysis. *Journal of Clinical Psychology, 74*(11), 1964–1979. https://doi.org/10.1002/jclp.22683

Ladany, N., Hill, C. E., Corbett, M. M., & Nutt, E. A. (1996). Nature, extent, and importance of what psychotherapy trainees do not disclose to their supervisors. *Journal of Counseling Psychology, 43*, 10–24. https://doi.org/10.1037/0022-0167.43.1.10

Lambert, M. J. (2010). *Prevention of treatment failure: The use of measuring, monitoring, and feedback in clinical practice.* American Psychological Association. https://doi.org/10.1037/12141-000

Lambert, M. J., Kahler, M., Harmon, C., Burlingame, G. M., Shimokawa, K., & White, M. M. (2013). *Administration and scoring manual: Outcome Questionnaire OQ®-45.2.* OQMeasures.

Lambert, M. J., Whipple, J. L., & Kleinstäuber, M. (2019). Collecting and delivering client feedback. In J. C. Norcross & M. J. Lambert (Eds.), *Psychotherapy relationships that work: Vol. 1. Evidence-based therapist contributions* (3rd ed., p. 580). Oxford University Press. https://doi.org/10.1093/med-psych/9780190843953.003.0017

Lau, A. S. (2006). Making the case for selective and directed cultural adaptations of evidence-based treatments: Examples from parent training. *Clinical Psychology: Science and Practice, 13*(4), 295–310. https://doi.org/10.1111/j.1468-2850.2006.00042.x

Lazarus, A. A. (1971). Where do behavior therapists take their troubles? *Psychological Reports, 28*(2), 349–350. https://doi.org/10.2466/pr0.1971.28.2.349

Lazarus, A. A. (1993). Tailoring the therapeutic relationship, or being an authentic chameleon. *Psychotherapy: Theory, Research, Practice, Training, 30*(3), 404–407. https://doi.org/10.1037/0033-3204.30.3.404

Lazarus, A. A., & Lazarus, C. N. (1998). Clinical purposes of the Multimodal Life History Inventory. In G. P. Koocher, J. C. Norcross, & S. S. Hill III (Eds.), *Psychologists' desk reference* (pp. 15–22). Oxford University Press.

Leigh, A. (1998). *Referral and termination issues for counsellors.* SAGE. https://doi.org/10.4135/9781446279793

Leon, S. C., Martinovich, Z., Lutz, W., & Lyons, J. S. (2005). The effect of therapist experience on psychotherapy outcomes. *Clinical Psychology & Psychotherapy, 12*(6), 417–426. https://doi.org/10.1002/cpp.473

Leotti, L. A., & Delgado, M. R. (2011). The inherent reward of choice. *Psychological Science, 22*(10), 1310–1318. https://doi.org/10.1177/0956797611417005

Levitt, H. M., Pomerville, A., & Surace, F. I. (2016). A qualitative meta-analysis examining clients' experiences of psychotherapy: A new agenda. *Psychological Bulletin, 142*(8), 801–830. https://doi.org/10.1037/bul0000057

Lichtenstein, S., & Slovic, P. (Eds.). (2006). *The construction of preference.* Cambridge University Press. https://doi.org/10.1017/CBO9780511618031

Lindhiem, O., Bennett, C. B., Trentacosta, C. J., & McLear, C. (2014). Client preferences affect treatment satisfaction, completion, and clinical outcome: A meta-analysis. *Clinical Psychology Review, 34*(6), 506–517. https://doi.org/10.1016/j.cpr.2014.06.002

Makoul, G., & Clayman, M. L. (2006). An integrative model of shared decision making in medical encounters. *Patient Education and Counseling, 60*(3), 301–312. https://doi.org/10.1016/j.pec.2005.06.010

Mathie, R. T., Ramparsad, N., Legg, L. A., Clausen, J., Moss, S., Davidson, J. R. T., Messow, C. M., & McConnachie, A. (2017). Randomised, double-blind, placebo-controlled trials of non-individualised homeopathic treatment: Systematic review and meta-analysis. *Systematic Reviews, 6*(1), 63. https://doi.org/10.1186/s13643-017-0445-3

Mazzucchelli, T. G., & Sanders, M. R. (2010). Facilitating practitioner flexibility within an empirically supported intervention: Lessons for a system of parenting support. *Clinical Psychology: Science and Practice, 17*(3), 238–252. https://doi.org/10.1111/j.1468-2850.2010.01215.x

McClelland, D. C., Koestner, R., & Weinberger, J. (1989). How do self-attributed and implicit motives differ? *Psychological Review, 96*(4), 690–702. https://doi.org/10.1037/0033-295X.96.4.690

McCullough, J. P., Jr. (2006). *Treating chronic depression with disciplined personal involvement: Cognitive behavioural analysis system of psychotherapy (CBASP)*. Springer. https://doi.org/10.1007/978-0-387-31066-4

McHugh, R. K., Whitton, S. W., Peckham, A. D., Welge, J. A., & Otto, M. W. (2013). Patient preference for psychological vs pharmacologic treatment of psychiatric disorders: A meta-analytic review. *The Journal of Clinical Psychiatry, 74*(6), 595–602. https://doi.org/10.4088/JCP.12r07757

McLeod, J. (2012). What do clients want from therapy? A practice-friendly review of research into client preferences. *European Journal of Psychotherapy and Counselling, 14*(1), 19–32. https://doi.org/10.1080/13642537.2012.652390

McLeod, J., & McLeod, J. (2016). Assessment and formulation in pluralistic counselling and psychotherapy. In M. Cooper & W. Dryden (Eds.), *Handbook of pluralistic counselling and psychotherapy* (pp. 15–27). SAGE.

McNeill, B. W., & Stoltenberg, C. D. (2016). *Supervision essentials for the integrative developmental model*. American Psychological Association. https://doi.org/10.1037/14858-000

Means, B., Toyama, Y., Murphy, R., & Baki, M. (2013). The effectiveness of online and blended learning: A meta-analysis of the empirical literature. *Teachers College Record, 115*(3), 1–47. https://www.tcrecord.org/library/content.asp?contentid=16882

Merriam-Webster. (n.d.). *Merriam-Webster.com dictionary*. Retrieved October 30, 2020, from https://www.merriam-webster.com/dictionary/preference

Metz, A. (2015). *Implementation brief: The potential of co-creation in implementation science*. nirn.fpg.unc.edu/sites/nirn.fpg.unc.edu/files/resources/NIRN-Metz-ImplementationBreif-CoCreation.pdf

Meyer, O. L., & Zane, N. (2013). The influence of race and ethnicity in clients' experiences of mental health treatment. *Journal of Community Psychology, 41*(7), 884–901. https://doi.org/10.1002/jcop.21580

Miller, S. D., Duncan, B. L., & Johnson, L. (2002). *The Session Rating Scale*. https://scottdmiller.com/wp-content/uploads/documents/SessionRatingScale-JBTv3n1.pdf

Miller, S. D., Hubble, M. A., & Chow, D. (2019). *Better results: Using deliberate practice to improve therapeutic effectiveness*. American Psychological Association.

Morán-Sánchez, I., Gómez-Vallés, P., Bernal-López, M. Á., & Pérez-Cárceles, M. D. (2019). Shared decision-making in outpatients with mental disorders: Patients' preferences and associated factors. *Journal of Evaluation in Clinical Practice, 25*(6), 1200–1209. https://doi.org/10.1111/jep.13246

Moskowitz, S. A., & Rupert, P. A. (1983). Conflict resolution within the supervisory relationship. *Professional Psychology: Research and Practice, 14*(5), 632–641. https://doi.org/10.1037/0735-7028.14.5.632

Mullen, B., Atkins, J. L., Champion, D. S., Edwards, C., Hardy, D., Story, J. E., & Vanderklok, M. (1985). The false consensus effect: A meta-analysis of 115 hypothesis tests. *Journal of Experimental Social Psychology, 21*(3), 262–283. https://doi.org/10.1016/0022-1031(85)90020-4

Nathan, P. E., & Gorman, J. M. (Eds.). (2015). *A guide to treatments that work* (4th ed.). Oxford University Press. https://doi.org/10.1093/med:psych/9780195304145.001.0001

National Health Service. (2016). *The five year forward view for mental health.* https://www.england.nhs.uk/wp-content/uploads/2016/02/Mental-Health-Taskforce-FYFV-final.pdf

National Implementation Research Network. (2005). *Implementation research: A synthesis of the literature.* https://nirn.fpg.unc.edu/resources/implementation-research-synthesis-literature

National Institute of Mental Health. (2015). *NIMH strategic plan for research* (NIH Publication No. 02-2650). https://www.nimh.nih.gov/about/strategic-planning-reports/index.shtml

Nelson, M. L., & Friedlander, M. L. (2001). A close look at conflictual supervisory relationships: The trainee's perspective. *Journal of Counseling Psychology, 48*(4), 384–395. https://doi.org/10.1037/0022-0167.48.4.384

NHS Centre for Reviews and Dissemination. (1999). Getting evidence into practice. *Effective Health Care, 5*(1), 1–16.

Norcross, J. C. (2005). The psychotherapist's own psychotherapy: Educating and developing psychologists. *American Psychologist, 60*(8), 840–850. https://doi.org/10.1037/0003-066X.60.8.840

Norcross, J. C., & Beutler, L. E. (2014). Evidence-based relationships and responsiveness for depression and substance abuse. In D. H. Barlow (Ed.), *Clinical handbook of psychological disorders* (5th ed., pp. 617–639). Guilford Press.

Norcross, J. C., Campbell, L. M., Grohol, J. M., Santrock, J. W., Selagea, F., & Sommer, R. (2013). *Self-help that works: Resources to improve emotional health and strengthen relationships* (4th ed.). Oxford University Press.

Norcross, J. C., & Goldfried, M. R. (Eds.). (2019). *Handbook of psychotherapy integration* (3rd ed.). Oxford University Press.

Norcross, J. C., & Halgin, R. P. (1997). Integrative approaches to psychotherapy supervision. In C. E. Watkins (Ed.), *Handbook of psychotherapy supervision* (pp. 203–222). Wiley.

Norcross, J. C., Hogan, T. P., Koocher, G. P., & Maggio, L. A. (2017). *Clinician's guide to evidence-based practices: Behavioral health and addictions*

(2nd ed.). Oxford University Press. https://doi.org/10.1093/med:psych/9780190621933.001.0001

Norcross, J. C., Koocher, G. P., & Garofalo, A. (2006). Discredited psychological treatments and tests: A Delphi poll. *Professional Psychology: Research and Practice, 37*(5), 515–522. https://doi.org/10.1037/0735-7028.37.5.515

Norcross, J. C., & Lambert, M. J. (Eds.). (2019). *Psychotherapy relationships that work: Volume 1. Evidence-based therapist contributions* (3rd ed.). Oxford University Press.

Norcross, J. C., & Popple, L. M. (2017). *Supervision essentials for integrative psychotherapy*. American Psychological Association. https://doi.org/10.1037/15967-000

Norcross, J. C., VandenBos, G. R., & Freedheim, D. K. (Eds.). (2016). *APA handbook of clinical psychology*. American Psychological Association.

Norcross, J. C., & Wampold, B. E. (2018). A new therapy for each patient: Evidence-based relationships and responsiveness. *Journal of Clinical Psychology, 74*(11), 1889–1906. https://doi.org/10.1002/jclp.22678

Norcross, J. C., & Wampold, B. E. (Eds.). (2019). *Psychotherapy relationships that work: Volume 2. Evidence-based therapist responsiveness* (3rd ed.). Oxford University Press.

Oldham, M., Kellett, S., Miles, E., & Sheeran, P. (2012). Interventions to increase attendance at psychotherapy: A meta-analysis of randomized controlled trials. *Journal of Consulting and Clinical Psychology, 80*(5), 928–939. https://doi.org/10.1037/a0029630

Orlinsky, D. E. (1989). Researchers' images of psychotherapy: Their origins and influence on research. *Clinical Psychology Review, 9*(4), 413–441. https://doi.org/10.1016/0272-7358(89)90002-0

Orlinsky, D. E., & Rønnestad, M. H. (2005). *How psychotherapists develop: A study of therapeutic work and professional growth*. American Psychological Association. https://doi.org/10.1037/11157-000

Orlinsky, D. E., Rønnestad, M. H., & Willutzki, U. (2004). Fifty years of psychotherapy process-outcome research: Continuity and change. In M. J. Lambert (Ed.), *Bergin and Garfield's handbook of psychotherapy and behavior change* (5th ed., pp. 307–389). Wiley.

Orwell, G. (2005). *Why I write*. Gangrel. (Original work published 1946)

Osler, W. (1906). *Aequanimatas*. McGraw-Hill.

Papayianni, F., & Cooper, M. (2018). Metatherapeutic communication: An exploratory analysis of therapist-reported moments of dialogue regarding the nature of the therapeutic work. *British Journal of Guidance & Counselling, 46*(2), 173–184. https://doi.org/10.1080/03069885.2017.1305098

Patel, S. R., Bakken, S., & Ruland, C. (2008). Recent advances in shared decision making for mental health. *Current Opinion in Psychiatry, 21*(6), 606–612. https://doi.org/10.1097/YCO.0b013e32830eb6b4

Paul, G. L. (1967). Strategy of outcome research in psychotherapy. *Journal of Consulting Psychology, 31*(2), 109–118. https://doi.org/10.1037/h0024436

Perez Jolles, M., Richmond, J., & Thomas, K. C. (2019). Minority patient preferences, barriers, and facilitators for shared decision-making with health care providers in the USA: A systematic review. *Patient Education and Counseling,* *102*(7), 1251–1262. https://doi.org/10.1016/j.pec.2019.02.003

Pipher, M. B. (1994). *Reviving Ophelia.* Putnam.

Powers, W. T. (1973). *Behaviour: The control of perception.* Aldine.

Preference Collaborative Review Group, & McPherson. (2009). Patients' preferences within randomised trials: Systematic review and patient level meta-analysis. *BMJ: British Medical Journal, 338*(7686), 85–88. https://www.jstor.org/stable/20511747

Prescott, D. S., Maeschalck, C. L., & Miller, S. D. (Eds.). (2017). *Feedback-informed treatment in clinical practice: Reaching for excellence.* American Psychological Association. https://doi.org/10.1037/0000039-000

Prochaska, J. O., DiClemente, C. C., & Norcross, J. C. (1992). In search of how people change: Applications to addictive behaviors. *American Psychologist, 47*(9), 1102–1114. https://doi.org/10.1037/0003-066X.47.9.1102

Prochaska, J. O., & Norcross, J. C. (2018). *Systems of psychotherapy: A transtheoretical analysis* (9th ed.). Oxford University Press.

Prochaska, J. O., Norcross, J. C., & Saul, S. F. (2020). Generating psychotherapy breakthroughs: Transtheoretical strategies from population health psychology. *American Psychologist, 75*(7), 996–1010. https://doi.org/10.1037/amp0000568

Rakovshik, S. G., McManus, F., Vazquez-Montes, M., Muse, K., & Ougrin, D. (2016). Is supervision necessary? Examining the effects of internet-based CBT training with and without supervision. *Journal of Consulting and Clinical Psychology, 84*(3), 191–199. https://doi.org/10.1037/ccp0000079

Rennie, D. L. (1994). Clients' deference in psychotherapy. *Journal of Counseling Psychology, 41*(4), 427–437. https://doi.org/10.1037/0022-0167.41.4.427

Richmond, H., Copsey, B., Hall, A. M., Davies, D., & Lamb, S. E. (2017). A systematic review and meta-analysis of online versus alternative methods for training licensed health care professionals to deliver clinical interventions. *BMC Medical Education, 17*(1), 227. https://doi.org/10.1186/s12909-017-1047-4

Riedel-Heller, S. G., Matschinger, H., & Angermeyer, M. C. (2005). Mental disorders—who and what might help? Help-seeking and treatment preferences of the lay public. *Social Psychiatry and Psychiatric Epidemiology, 40*(2), 167–174. https://doi.org/10.1007/s00127-005-0863-8

Rose, J. P., Geers, A. L., Rasinski, H. M., & Fowler, S. L. (2012). Choice and placebo expectation effects in the context of pain analgesia. *Journal of Behavioral Medicine, 35*(4), 462–470. https://doi.org/10.1007/s10865-011-9374-0

Ross, L., Greene, D., & House, P. (1977). The "false consensus effect": An egocentric bias in social perception and attribution processes. *Journal of Experimental Social Psychology, 13*(3), 279–301. https://doi.org/10.1016/0022-1031(77)90049-X

Rousmaniere, T., Goodyear, R. K., Miller, S. D., & Wampold, B. E. (Eds.). (2017). *The cycle of excellence: Using deliberate practice to improve supervision and training*. Wiley. https://doi.org/10.1002/9781119165590

Sackett, D. L., Straus, S. E., Richardson, W. S., Rosenberg, W., & Haynes, R. B. (2000). *Evidence-based medicine: How to practice and teach EBM* (2nd ed.). Churchill-Livingstone.

Safran, J. D., & Muran, J. C. (2000). Resolving therapeutic alliance ruptures: Diversity and integration. *Journal of Clinical Psychology, 56*(2), 233–243. https://doi.org/10.1002/(SICI)1097-4679(200002)56:2<233::AID-JCLP9>3.0.CO;2-3

Safran, J. D., Muran, J. C., Samstag, L. W., & Stevens, C. (2002). Repairing alliance ruptures. In J. C. Norcross (Ed.), *Psychotherapy relationships that work* (pp. 235–254). Oxford University Press.

Sandell, R., Clinton, D., Frövenholt, J., & Bragesjö, M. (2011). Credibility clusters, preferences, and helpfulness beliefs for specific forms of psychotherapy. *Psychology and Psychotherapy: Theory, Research and Practice, 84*(4), 425–441. https://doi.org/10.1111/j.2044-8341.2010.02010.x

SANE. (2014). *Living with schizophrenia: People's experience of the condition.* http://www.sane.org.uk/uploads/living-with-schizophrenia-final-uk_am_0414_0121_vcertification_1-2.pdf

Shang, A., Huwiler-Müntener, K., Nartey, L., Jüni, P., Dörig, S., Sterne, J. A., Pewsner, D., & Egger, M. (2005). Are the clinical effects of homoeopathy placebo effects? Comparative study of placebo-controlled trials of homoeopathy and allopathy. *The Lancet, 366*(9487), 726–732. https://doi.org/10.1016/S0140-6736(05)67177-2

Sharot, T., De Martino, B., & Dolan, R. J. (2009). How choice reveals and shapes expected hedonic outcome. *The Journal of Neuroscience, 29*(12), 3760–3765. https://doi.org/10.1523/JNEUROSCI.4972-08.2009

Simiola, V., Ellis, A. E., Thompson, R., Schnurr, P. P., & Cook, J. M. (2019). Provider perspectives on choosing prolonged exposure of cognitive processing therapy for PTSD: A national investigation of VA residential treatment providers. *Practice Innovations, 4*(3), 194–203. https://doi.org/10.1037/pri0000091

Soto, A., Smith, T. B., Griner, D., Domenech Rodríguez, M., & Bernal, G. (2018). Cultural adaptations and therapist multicultural competence: Two meta-analytic reviews. *Journal of Clinical Psychology, 74*(11), 1907–1923. https://doi.org/10.1002/jclp.22679

Spitzer, R. L., Kroenke, K., Williams, J. B., & Patient Health Questionnaire Primary Care Study Group. (1999). Validation and utility of a self-report version of PRIME-MD: The PHQ primary care study. *JAMA, 282*(18), 1737–1744. https://doi.org/10.1001/jama.282.18.1737

Stacey, D., Légaré, F., Col, N. F., Bennett, C. L., Barry, M. J., Eden, K. B., Holmes-Rovner, M., Llewellyn-Thomas, H., Lyddiatt, A., Thomson, R., Trevena, L., & Wu, J. H. C. (2014). Decision aids for people facing health treatment or screening decisions. *Cochrane Database of Systematic Reviews*. https://doi.org/10.1002/14651858.CD001431.pub4

Stein, B. D., Celedonia, K. L., Swartz, H. A., DeRosier, M. E., Sorbero, M. J., Brindley, R. A., Burns, R. M., Dick, A. W., & Frank, E. (2015). Implementing a web-based intervention to train community clinicians in an evidence-based psychotherapy: A pilot study. *Psychiatric Services*, *66*(9), 988–991. https://doi.org/10.1176/appi.ps.201400318

Stewart, T. J., Swift, J. K., Freitas-Murrell, B. N., & Whipple, J. L. (2013). Preferences for mental health treatment options among Alaska Native college students. *American Indian and Alaska Native Mental Health Research*, *20*(3), 59–78. https://doi.org/10.5820/aian.2003.2013.59

Stiles, W. B., Honos-Webb, L., & Surko, M. (1998). Responsiveness in psychotherapy. *Clinical Psychology: Science and Practice*, *5*(4), 439–458. https://doi.org/10.1111/j.1468-2850.1998.tb00166.x

Stovell, D., Morrison, A. P., Panayiotou, M., & Hutton, P. (2016). Shared treatment decision-making and empowerment-related outcomes in psychosis: Systematic review and meta-analysis. *The British Journal of Psychiatry*, *209*(1), 23–28. https://doi.org/10.1192/bjp.bp.114.158931

Sue, D. W., Sue, S., Neville, H. A., & Smith, L. (2019). *Counseling the culturally diverse: Theory and practice* (8th ed.). Wiley.

Swift, J. K., & Callahan, J. L. (2010). A comparison of client preferences for intervention empirical support versus common therapy variables. *Journal of Clinical Psychology*, *66*(12), 1217–1231. https://doi.org/10.1002/jclp.20720

Swift, J. K., Callahan, J. L., Cooper, M., & Parkin, S. R. (2018). The impact of accommodating client preference in psychotherapy: A meta-analysis. *Journal of Clinical Psychology*, *74*(11), 1924–1937. https://doi.org/10.1002/jclp.22680

Swift, J. K., Callahan, J. L., Cooper, M., & Parkin, S. R. (2019). Preferences. In J. C. Norcross & B. E. Wampold (Eds.), *Psychotherapy relationships that work: Vol. 2. Evidence-based therapist responsiveness* (3rd ed., p. 157). Oxford University. https://doi.org/10.1093/med-psych/9780190843960.003.0006

Swift, J. K., Callahan, J. L., Ivanovic, M., & Kominiak, N. (2013). Further examination of the psychotherapy preference effect: A meta-regression analysis. *Journal of Psychotherapy Integration*, *23*(2), 134–145. https://doi.org/10.1037/a0031423

Swift, J. K., Callahan, J. L., Tompkins, K. A., Connor, D. R., & Dunn, R. (2015). A delay-discounting measure of preference for racial/ethnic matching in psychotherapy. *Psychotherapy*, *52*(3), 315–320. https://doi.org/10.1037/pst0000019

Swift, J. K., Callahan, J. L., & Vollmer, B. M. (2011). Preferences. *Journal of Clinical Psychology*, *67*(2), 155–165. https://doi.org/10.1002/jclp.20759

Swift, J. K., & Greenberg, R. P. (2014). A treatment by disorder meta-analysis of dropout from psychotherapy. *Journal of Psychotherapy Integration*, *24*(3), 193–207. https://doi.org/10.1037/a0037512

Swift, J. K., & Greenberg, R. P. (2015). *Premature termination in psychotherapy: Strategies for engaging clients and improving outcomes.* American Psychological Association. https://doi.org/10.1037/14469-000

Tasca, G. A., Sylvestre, J., Balfour, L., Chyurlia, L., Evans, J., Fortin-Langelier, B., Francis, K., Gandhi, J., Huehn, L., Hunsley, J., Joyce, A. S., Kinley, J., Koszycki, D., Leszcz, M., Lybanon-Daigle, V., Mercer, D., Ogrodniczuk, J. S., Presniak, M., Ravitz, P., . . . Wilson, B. (2015). What clinicians want: Findings from a psychotherapy practice research network survey. *Psychotherapy, 52*(1), 1–11. https://doi.org/10.1037/a0038252

Thoma, N. C., & Cecero, J. J. (2009). Is integrative use of techniques in psychotherapy the exception or the rule? Results of a national survey of doctoral-level practitioners. *Psychotherapy, 46*(4), 405–417. https://doi.org/10.1037/a0017900

Thoreau, H. D. (1854). *Walden.* Princeton University Press.

Thrash, T. M., Maruskin, L. A., & Martin, C. C. (2012). Implicit-explicit motive congruence. In R. M. Ryan (Ed.), *The Oxford handbook of human motivation* (pp. 141–156). Oxford University Press.

Tompkins, K. A., Swift, J. K., & Callahan, J. L. (2013). Working with clients by incorporating their preferences. *Psychotherapy, 50*(3), 279–283. https://doi.org/10.1037/a0032031

Tompkins, K. A., Swift, J. K., Rousmaniere, T. G., & Whipple, J. L. (2017). The relationship between clients' depression etiological beliefs and psychotherapy orientation preferences, expectations, and credibility beliefs. *Psychotherapy, 54*(2), 201–206. https://doi.org/10.1037/pst0000070

Tracey, T. J. G., Wampold, B. E., Lichtenberg, J. W., & Goodyear, R. K. (2014). Expertise in psychotherapy: An elusive goal? *American Psychologist, 69*(3), 218–229. https://doi.org/10.1037/a0035099

Trusty, W. T., Penix, E. A., Dimmick, A. A., & Swift, J. K. (2019). Shared decision-making in mental and behavioural health interventions. *Journal of Evaluation in Clinical Practice, 25*(6), 1210–1216. https://doi.org/10.1111/jep.13255

Vermes, C., & Cooper, M. (2020). *C-NIP data* [Unpublished raw data].

Vollmer, B., Grote, J., Lange, R., & Walker, C. (2009). A therapy preferences interview: Empowering clients by offering choices. *Psychotherapy Bulletin, 44*(2), 33–37.

Walfish, S., McAlister, B., O'Donnell, P., & Lambert, M. J. (2012). An investigation of self-assessment bias in mental health providers. *Psychological Reports, 110*(2), 639–644. https://doi.org/10.2466/02.07.17.PR0.110.2.639-644

Walfish, S., & Zimmerman, J. (2013). Making good referrals. In G. P. Koocher, J. C. Norcross, & B. A. Greene (Eds.), *Psychologists' desk reference* (3rd ed., pp. 649–654). Oxford University Press. https://doi.org/10.1093/med:psych/9780199845491.003.0124

Wallace, K., & Cooper, M. (2015). Development of supervision personalisation forms: A qualitative study of the dimensions along which supervisors' practices vary. *Counselling & Psychotherapy Research, 15*(1), 31–40. https://doi.org/10.1002/capr.12001

Walsh, L. M., Roddy, M. K., Scott, K., Lewis, C. C., & Jensen-Doss, A. (2019). A meta-analysis of the effect of therapist experience on outcomes for clients with internalizing disorders. *Psychotherapy Research, 29*(7), 846–859. https://doi.org/10.1080/10503307.2018.1469802

Wampold, B. E., & Imel, Z. (2015). *The great psychotherapy debate* (2nd ed.). Erlbaum. https://doi.org/10.4324/9780203582015

Wiggins, J. S. (1979). A psychological taxonomy of trait-descriptive terms: The interpersonal domain. *Journal of Personality and Social Psychology, 37*(3), 395–412. https://doi.org/10.1037/0022-3514.37.3.395

Williams, R., Farquharson, L., Palmer, L., Bassett, P., Clarke, J., Clark, D. M., & Crawford, M. J. (2016). Patient preference in psychological treatment and associations with self-reported outcome: National cross-sectional survey in England and Wales. *BMC Psychiatry, 16*. https://doi.org/10.1186/s12888-015-0702-8

Windle, E., Tee, H., Sabitova, A., Jovanovic, N., Priebe, S., & Carr, C. (2019). Association of patient treatment preference with dropout and clinical outcomes in adult psychosocial mental health interventions. *JAMA Psychiatry, 77*(3), 294–302. https://doi.org/10.1001/jamapsychiatry.2019.3750

Winter, S. E., & Barber, J. P. (2013). Should treatment for depression be based more on patient preference? *Patient Preference and Adherence, 7*, 1047–1057. https://doi.org/10.2147/PPA.S52746

Wolitzky, D. L. (2011). Psychoanalytic theories of psychotherapy. In J. C. Norcross, G. R. VandenBos, & D. K. Freedheim (Eds.), *History of psychotherapy* (2nd ed., pp. 65–100). American Psychological Association. https://doi.org/10.1037/12353-003

World Health Organization. (2011). *Mental health atlas 2011.* https://www.who.int/mental_health/publications/mental_health_atlas_2011/en/

Wyatt, K. D., List, B., Brinkman, W. B., Prutsky Lopez, G., Asi, N., Erwin, P., Wang, Z., Domecq Garces, J. P., Montori, V. M., & LeBlanc, A. (2015). Shared decision making in pediatrics: A systematic review and meta-analysis. *Academic Pediatrics, 15*(6), 573–583. https://doi.org/10.1016/j.acap.2015.03.011

Yulish, N. E., Goldberg, S. B., Frost, N. D., Abbas, M., Oleen-Junk, N. A., Kring, M., Chin, M. Y., Raines, C. R., Soma, C. S., & Wampold, B. E. (2017). The importance of problem-focused treatments: A meta-analysis of anxiety treatments. *Psychotherapy, 54*(4), 321–338. https://doi.org/10.1037/pst0000144

Zilcha-Mano, S. (2017). Is the alliance really therapeutic? Revisiting this question in light of recent methodological advances. *American Psychologist, 72*(4), 311–325. https://doi.org/10.1037/a0040435

Index

About the Authors

John C. Norcross, PhD, ABPP, is Distinguished Professor and Chair of psychology at the University of Scranton, clinical professor of psychiatry at SUNY Upstate Medical University, and a board-certified clinical psychologist. Dr. Norcross has cowritten or edited 22 books, including the five-volume *APA Handbook of Clinical Psychology*; *Psychotherapy Relationships That Work*; *Handbook of Psychotherapy Integration*; *Insider's Guide to Graduate Programs in Clinical and Counseling Psychology*; and *Systems of Psychotherapy: A Transtheoretical Analysis*, now in its ninth edition. Dr. Norcross has been elected president of the American Psychological Association (APA) Society of Clinical Psychology, the APA Society for the Advancement of Psychotherapy, the International Society of Clinical Psychology, and the Society for the Exploration of Psychotherapy Integration. He edited the *Journal of Clinical Psychology* for a decade and has been on the editorial boards of a dozen journals. Dr. Norcross has received multiple professional awards, such as APA's Distinguished Career Contributions to Education and Training in Psychology award, Pennsylvania Professor of the Year from the Carnegie Foundation, and election to the National Academies of Practice. He has conducted workshops and lectures in 30 countries.

Mick Cooper, DPhil, is Professor of counselling psychology at the University of Roehampton, where he directs the Centre for Research in Social and Psychological Transformation (CREST). Dr. Cooper is a chartered psychologist, a United Kingdom Council for Psychotherapy–registered existential psychotherapist, and a fellow of the British Association for Counselling and Psychotherapy. He is author and editor of multiple texts on person-centered, existential, and relational approaches to therapy, including *Working at Relational Depth in Counselling and Psychotherapy*; *Existential Therapies*; and

Integrating Counselling and Psychotherapy: Directionality, Synergy, and Social Change. Dr. Cooper has led a series of research studies—both qualitative and quantitative—exploring the processes and outcomes of humanistic counseling with young people and has published in a range of leading international journals. He is the father of four children and lives in Brighton on the south coast of England.